Imposter Syndrome: Silencing the Self-Doubt Within the Workplace

By Dr. Joshan A. Flowers, DSL

Published by:

Pine Book Writing

www.PineBookWriting.com

R-10225 Yonge St Suite #250, Richmond Hill, ON L4C 3B2, Canada.

Table of Contents

In Loving Memory:

Christine Scott
Charles Tidwell
Ann Tidwell
Lewis Flowers Jr.
Donnell C. Flowers
Christine Flowers
James M. Banks
Cecilia Banks

Dedication

This book is dedicated to my children, Billah and Hadiyyah,
my husband, Ramni, and my grandmother Christine Scott,
who I know is very proud of me.

Acknowledgment

Firstly, I give all honor and glory to God. I am deeply grateful for God's continuous support in my emotional, mental, physical, spiritual, and intellectual well-being. It is through God's grace and mercy that I recognize the significance of completing this book.

Secondly, this wouldn't have been possible without my children and my niece in my life. I owe my success to them for being my biggest cheerleaders, always there to provide encouragement. They prayed and cheered me on throughout the journey to the finish line. Billah, Hadiyyah, and Gia, I love you all more than words could ever convey. I could never repay you for the love and support that each of you has shown while on this journey, but I can say, "Thank you!" Also, my husband Ramni, you are my anchor and have provided not only a safe space for me but a strong hug that I love.

Lastly, I would like to give a special thanks to Ms. Alva Anthony who fought for my selection into the United Air Force Bootstrap program while serving on Active Duty. She alone is the reason that I received my bachelor's degree. Thank you to my family: my mom, Jocelyn Flowers, my sister Jocelyn C. Flowers, my niece, Gia; my nephews, Jay and Devin, my uncles, Victor Flowers, Corneilus Flowers, and Dennis Flowers, my aunts Lorinda Givens and VFW Commander Post 311 Aretha Johnson-Spurlock, and lastly, my ROD Teajaii. With heartfelt gratitude and love, my family remains steadfast at my side, ever ready to uplift me and provide the strength and courage needed on this voyage through life.

Foreword

Every workplace has its own strengths and challenges that both build up and break down people on a daily occurrence. Whether you are someone who is just beginning your career or you are a seasoned veteran, imposter syndrome is indiscriminatory. The world of academia is no different and it is where my imposter syndrome was born. Having graduated from George Mason University with a bachelor's degree in government and international politics and a master's degree in public policy at the age of 22 there were plenty of voices, externally and internally, that made me question my own knowledge and self-worth. I was told I was too young, too ambitious, too careless, and too naivë to achieve all the things I set my sights on. However, what those who suffer from imposter syndrome do not know is that although it is through the words and actions of others that create our conditions, only we can restore and reinforce our true identities. And, that is the message and purpose of Dr. Flowers's words in this book.

Growing it was my parents who instilled in me the importance of practicing self-confidence and self-worth until it was unequivocally my truth. Whether it was on the playground, classroom, or in the office, my parents always told my brother and me to "do what is right and always be yourself, especially when no one is watching". Imposters syndrome is not born in people until others and challenging situations make them question who they are. Fortunately, my mother, Dr. Flowers, taught me and countless others on how to overcome such challenges, and she has finally accomplished her lifelong dream of wanting to share her expertise and insight with you, her readers. Dr. Flowers has been a mentor to those with varying degrees of experience since her time as a United States Air Force Master Sergeant. She has mentored career professionals, college students, and adolescent military children.

So, as you proceed to read through Dr. Flowers' chapters, please remember these two important notes from the author;

(1) no one is born with imposter syndrome, and (2) however patiently and unrelentingly persistent your imposter syndrome develops in your workplace, you have and will always have the ability to remind yourself that you are enough. Please enjoy and keep an open mind as you acquire lessons on how to silence your self-doubt within the workplace.

Hadiyyah Abdul-Jalaal

I am incredibly proud to introduce this book on imposter syndrome in the workspace, written by my amazing mom. Throughout her career, she has faced numerous challenges and obstacles, but she has always persevered and come out stronger on the other side. Her journey is a testament to the power of resilience and determination. In these pages, she shares her personal experiences and insights, offering a guiding light for all those who have ever felt like they don't belong or that their accomplishments are undeserved.

As I read through the chapters of this book, I couldn't help but be inspired by my mom's courage and vulnerability. She opens up about her own struggles with imposter syndrome, shedding light on the internal battles that so many of us face in the workplace. But this book is not just about her journey; it is a call to action for anyone who has ever doubted their abilities or felt like they were not good enough. Through her words, my mom encourages us all to embrace our strengths, celebrate our achievements, and recognize that we are not alone in our feelings of inadequacy.

To all those who may be reading this book and questioning their worth, I want you to know that you are not alone. Imposter syndrome is a common experience, and it does not define your capabilities or potential. My mom's story is a reminder that we are all capable of greatness, even in the face of self-doubt. So, as you embark on this journey through the pages of this book, I encourage you to embrace your unique talents, believe in yourself, and know that you have the power to overcome any challenge that comes your way. Let this book be your guide and your source of inspiration as you navigate the complexities of the modern workplace.

Billah Abdul-Jalaal
Owner of Elysian Health
Founder of Taking The First Step

Chapter 1
Understanding Imposter Syndrome

Do you often experience a persistent sense that your efforts are never quite sufficient, and self-doubt clings to you relentlessly? Have you ever caught yourself pondering thoughts like, "I'm a fraud," "I don't belong here," or "I'm not intelligent enough for this"? Despite a lengthy list of accomplishments, you still feel as if you're lagging behind others. Even when you're the most successful person in a room, self-satisfaction remains elusive. If this resonates with you, you might be struggling with Impostor Syndrome. You're not alone in this experience, as these thoughts are quite common, and when they persist, they are often indicative of imposter syndrome (IS). In the presence of imposter syndrome, individuals frequently face these recurring feelings or thoughts that they lack competence or fall short, even when evidence suggests otherwise. This self-doubt can have a significant impact on various aspects of life, but recognizing it is the first step towards overcoming it and embracing your true capabilities.

Imposter syndrome, imposter phenomenon or imposterism, is a psychological pattern in which an individual doubts their own skills, talents, and accomplishments and has a constant fear of being exposed as a fraud, despite evidence to the contrary. People experiencing imposter syndrome attribute their success to luck, timing, or other external factors rather than their own abilities and hard work. They feel as though they don't deserve the recognition and opportunities they've received, and they fear that others will eventually discover that they are not as competent as they appear.

Imposter syndrome can affect individuals in various aspects of their lives, including their careers, education, and personal relationships. It can lead to self-doubt, anxiety, and a reluctance to take on new challenges or opportunities, as people with imposter syndrome often underestimate their own capabilities.

It's important to note that imposter syndrome is a common experience and can affect people from all backgrounds and levels of achievement - it's not limited to a specific gender, age group, or profession. Overcoming imposter syndrome involves recognizing the feelings associated with it, challenging negative self-perceptions, and seeking support and feedback from others to gain a more accurate perspective of one's abilities and accomplishments.

Imposter syndrome - a psychological phenomenon that has a significant and far-reaching impact on individuals' lives. At its core, it undermines self-confidence and self-worth, sowing the seeds of self-doubt that often results in a hesitancy to embrace new opportunities or set ambitious goals. This chronic self-doubt also breeds a fear of failure, pushing those affected to avoid challenges and to set impossibly high standards for themselves, leading to the trap of perfectionism, which can cause chronic stress and even burnout.

The self-deprecating mindset associated with imposter syndrome can also exhibit an inability to accept praise and a vulnerability to mental health issues, such as anxiety and depression. In personal relationships, it can create strains as individuals struggle with the constant need to prove themselves or, in some cases, withdraw from social situations to avoid potential judgment.

Professionally, the effects of imposter syndrome can be particularly pronounced. Individuals may find that they shy away from seeking promotions, applying for new opportunities, or actively participating in the workplace because they believe they lack the qualifications or competence that are required. This sense of inadequacy can then hinder job performance and limit career advancement.

The effect of this permanent feeling of being an imposter can lead to work-related stress, impacting overall well-being and the ability to find satisfaction in one's personal and professional life. Overcoming imposter syndrome is not a straightforward task, but it involves acknowledging these feelings, seeking support, challenging negative thought patterns, and building self-confidence. Ultimately, it requires learning to accept one's achievements and believe in one's capabilities to break free from the chains of imposter syndrome and lead a more fulfilled and successful life.

CHARACTERISTICS OF IMPOSTER SYNDROME

Imposter syndrome can take on different forms, with individuals often exhibiting a mix of traits. Nevertheless, there are several common characteristics and behaviors frequently linked to imposter syndrome, including:

Self-Doubt: Constantly doubting your abilities and competence, even when you have clear evidence of your skills and accomplishments. This self-doubt acts like a constant internal critic, causing ongoing uncertainty and self-criticism. Even when you've achieved genuine success, you may still feel incapable and stuck in a cycle of doubt.

Perfectionism: Setting extremely high, often unachievable standards for oneself, leading to a fear of any imperfection or deviation from perfection. This means individuals place intense demands on themselves in multiple areas of their lives, like work, relationships, and personal goals. They become fixated on achieving flawless results in everything they do and see even the slightest mistake as unacceptable.

Overachievement: Overworking or constantly striving to excel in every task as a means to validate one's worth is another characteristic trait of impostor syndrome. Individuals with this trait often feel compelled to push themselves to their limits in order to prove their competence and value. They may take on an excessive workload, work long hours, or go to great lengths to achieve exceptional results in every endeavor.

Fear of Failure: An intense fear of making mistakes or experiencing failure, as it may confirm feelings of ineffectiveness, is a core component of impostor syndrome. People struggling with this trait are often consumed by the dread of getting things wrong or falling short of their own, often impossibly high, expectations. They view errors or failures not as opportunities for growth but as affirmations of their lack of competence.

Undermining Success: Downplaying or attributing personal achievements to external factors like luck, rather than acknowledging one's abilities and hard work, is a characteristic behavior associated with impostor syndrome. Individuals with this trait tend to minimize or disregard their accomplishments, as they believe that external factors, such as luck, timing, or the help of others, played a more significant role in their success than their own skills or efforts.

Difficulty Accepting Praise: Struggling to accept compliments or recognition for accomplishments and feeling uncomfortable when praised is a common behavior among individuals with impostor syndrome. This trait often manifests as discomfort or uneasiness when someone acknowledges their achievements or offers a compliment. They may deflect or downplay the praise, attributing their success to external factors or dismissing it as insincere.

Comparing to Others: Frequently comparing oneself to others and believing that everyone else is more competent or accomplished. Individuals with this trait engage in a relentless cycle of self-comparison, often perceiving their peers and colleagues as more capable, accomplished, or talented, regardless of the evidence to the contrary.

Discounting Achievements: Believing that personal achievements are not significant or important, even when they are, is a distinct trait associated with impostor syndrome. Individuals with this characteristic tend to downplay the value and impact of their accomplishments, dismissing their successes as inconsequential or attributing them to external factors.

Reluctance to Share: Hesitancy to share one's thoughts, ideas, or work, fueled by the fear of potential criticism or rejection, is a common behavior. With this trait, individuals often feel a reluctance to express themselves or showcase their work, fearing that it may not meet the perceived high standards of others or that they will face judgment. This hesitancy can hinder effective communication and collaboration, as individuals may hold back valuable contributions due to the fear of not measuring up. The fear of criticism or rejection reinforces the belief that their ideas or work are not valid or worthy of consideration.

Overwork and Burnout: Overextending oneself to prove competence, leading to exhaustion and burnout, is a common behavior associated with impostor syndrome. Individuals often feel compelled to go above and beyond in their efforts to demonstrate their capabilities, constantly striving to meet or exceed perceived expectations. This overextension may manifest as taking on an excessive workload, volunteering for numerous tasks, or consistently working long hours.

Seeking External Validation: Relying on external validation and seeking constant reassurance from others to feel competent is a notable behavior. Which frequently places a heavy reliance on the opinions and feedback of others to validate their sense of competence and worth. The individuals may constantly seek reassurance that their work is acceptable or that they are doing well, using external feedback as a means of validating their own abilities.

Procrastination: Delaying tasks due to the fear of not being able to complete them perfectly or to avoid potential criticism. You may experience a paralyzing fear that your work will not meet your own exceedingly high standards, leading to a reluctance to start or complete tasks. The desire for perfection can become a significant obstacle, as you may procrastinate to avoid the discomfort of potential imperfection or the perceived threat of criticism. This fear of not meeting self-imposed standards can be a significant source of stress and anxiety, hindering productivity and personal growth.

It's important to note that not everyone with imposter syndrome exhibits all of these traits, and the significance of these behaviors can vary from person to person. Recognizing these traits in oneself is an essential step toward addressing imposter syndrome and developing a healthier self-perception.

PSYCHOLOGICAL ASPECTS OF IMPOSTER SYNDROME

The psychological aspects of imposter syndrome are rooted in complex thought patterns and emotional responses that contribute to self-doubt and feelings of failure. Here are some key factors that underlie these psychological aspects:

High Standards: Imposter syndrome is closely tied to the psychological aspect of individuals setting exceptionally high standards for themselves. This inclination towards perfection creates a mental framework where any conflict from flawless performance is not only a deviation from personal expectations but also serves to fuel self-doubt.

Attribution Bias: There is a tendency to attribute success to external factors (luck, help from others) and failure to internal factors (personal incompetence). This biased thinking reinforces the belief that achievements are not a result of one's own abilities.

Social Comparison: Constantly comparing oneself to others, especially to those perceived as more successful or accomplished, can lead to a distorted self-perception. The focus on others' achievements can intensify feelings of inadequacy.

Impaired Self-Judgement: Individuals with imposter syndrome struggle to accurately evaluate their own competence. Positive feedback or evidence of success is often dismissed, while any negative feedback or mistakes are developed.

Fear of Evaluation: There's a heightened fear of being evaluated or judged by others. This fear can frighten individuals, preventing them from taking risks or putting themselves forward for opportunities.

Cultural and Societal Factors: External pressures, societal expectations, or cultural influences can contribute to imposter syndrome. For instance, individuals from marginalized groups may face additional challenges due to stereotype threat.

Early Life Experiences: Childhood experiences, such as excessive parental expectations or a lack of validation, can contribute to the development of imposter syndrome. Messages received during formative years can shape self-consciousness.

Fixed Mindset: Individuals with a fixed mindset believe that their abilities and intelligence are static traits. This mindset can lead to a fear of failure, which could result in blocking all the alternate options and only stubbornly focusing on one goal – you may feel like a complete failure when you're unable to achieve that.

Overgeneralization: An isolated failure or mistake is often generalized to the belief that one is a complete failure. This cognitive distortion strengthens feelings of inadequacy.

Understanding these psychological aspects is crucial for addressing imposter syndrome. Therapy, self-reflection, and cognitive-behavioral interventions are common approaches to challenge and reframe these negative thought patterns, fostering a more realistic and positive self-concept.

IMPOSTER SYNDROME IS IN PROFESSIONAL SETTINGS

Imposter syndrome is a widely recognized phenomenon, and numerous studies have explored its prevalence in professional settings. It's important to note that the occurrence can vary across industries, occupations, and demographics. Here are some key findings:

General Prevalence: Research from the International Journal of Behavioral Science suggests that up to 70% of individuals experience imposter syndrome at some point in their lives. This high prevalence indicates that a significant majority of people, at different stages in their personal and professional journeys, struggle with feelings of insecurity and self-doubt linked to imposter syndrome.

Occupational Differences: Research suggests that certain professions may have higher rates of imposter syndrome. For example, individuals in creative fields, academia, and healthcare are likely to experience imposter feelings. In such fields, the constant quest for innovation and originality can create a feeling of not measuring up. Academia's competitive nature may develop feelings of intellectual lack. Similarly, healthcare professionals dealing with complex and high-stakes situations may be more prone to questioning their abilities.

Academic Settings: Studies often focus on academic or educational settings. For instance, a study published in the Journal of Vocational Behavior found that impostor syndrome is prevalent among graduate students, with around 47% reporting moderate to intense feelings of imposterism.

Gender Disparities: Research has explored gender differences in experiencing imposter syndrome. Some studies suggest that women may be more likely to report experiencing impostor syndrome, possibly due to societal expectations and stereotypes about women's capabilities. However, it's essential to emphasize that impostor syndrome is not limited to any gender; men also experience these feelings.

Impact on Career Development: A study published in the Journal of Career Development found that imposter syndrome is negatively associated with career development and satisfaction. Individuals experiencing imposter feelings may be less likely to pursue career advancement opportunities.

Global Perspectives: Imposter syndrome is not limited to specific cultures or regions. Research has shown its presence in various countries, highlighting its global nature. Cultural expectations and societal norms can influence the manifestation of impostor feelings.

Age Groups: While much research focuses on adults, imposter syndrome can also affect younger individuals. Studies have explored its popularity among students and young professionals, discovering its impact on educational and career paths.

It's worth noting that imposter syndrome is a subjective experience, and self-reporting in studies plays a significant role. The stigma associated with admitting such feelings may also result in under-reporting. Despite these challenges, the consistent findings across diverse studies highlight the widespread nature of imposter syndrome in professional settings. Awareness of it is crucial for organizations and individuals to implement strategies that promote a supportive and affirming workplace culture.

Imposter syndrome is widely acknowledged as a massive issue in today's workplace, affecting a substantial portion of the workforce. Research consistently indicates that estimates of individuals experiencing imposter feelings range from 30% to 70%, emphasizing its common occurrence. This phenomenon is not confined to specific industries, as evidence of its impact extends across a broad spectrum, encompassing technology, healthcare, finance, academia, engineering, marketing, the arts, and various other sectors. While individuals of all genders experience imposter syndrome, some studies suggest that women may be more likely to report these feelings, highlighting the influence of gender dynamics in the workplace. This issue goes beyond global borders, as research conducted in diverse cultural contexts underlines its universal nature.

Additionally, workplace culture plays a crucial role, with environments fostering open communication and psychological safety better positioned to address imposters' feelings. The rise of remote work has introduced new challenges related to imposter syndrome, emphasizing the importance of initiatives promoting mental well-being and confidence in the evolving professional landscape. Recognizing the widespread nature of imposter syndrome is vital for organizations to implement strategies that cultivate supportive workplace cultures and prioritize employee mental health and career development.

Chapter 2
Recognizing Imposter Syndrome in Yourself

Now that you're familiar with Imposter Syndrome, let's start by identifying its subtle signs and symptoms that can easily slip by unnoticed. It's important to catch these hints because they might not be obvious. Imposter Syndrome shows up in different ways, and understanding its more hidden symptoms is crucial. So, we'll examine these subtle cues that could indicate Imposter Syndrome, bringing attention to aspects that might be easily overlooked.

If you have Imposter Syndrome, you might think you don't deserve success. You could be telling yourself, "I may seem more competent than I truly am," or "I'm worried my colleagues will find out how little I really know." The fear of being exposed and having others discover your perceived inadequacy is a common aspect. The ongoing sense that you're barely avoiding a professional disaster repeatedly can lead to a constant feeling of stress and anxiety. This can negatively impact all aspects of your work and relationships.

However, perceiving yourself as an imposter might tend to credit your accomplishments to luck. Thoughts like, "I happened to be in the right place at the right time," or "That was just a fluke," could be running through your mind. These thoughts indicate a fear that you won't be able to replicate your success in the future. They speak to a deep-seated belief that your achievements have little to do with your actual abilities. This mindset can create a sense of insecurity about your skills and competence, impacting your confidence in taking on future challenges. It's important to recognize these thoughts and work towards acknowledging your own capabilities.

If you experience Imposter Syndrome, you might tend to

downplay your achievements, thinking you're nothing special. You may tell yourself, "Oh, that was nothing. I'm sure my teammate could have done the same thing," or "I don't bring anything unique to the company that no one else could." Interestingly, studies reveal that individuals who strongly feel the effects of Imposter Syndrome often hold multiple advanced degrees and boast proven track records. Despite these accomplishments, the belief that your contributions are ordinary or easily replicable may hinder you from recognizing and embracing your individual strengths. It's important to acknowledge your unique abilities and contributions to overcome the challenges posed by Imposter Syndrome.

While struggling with Imposter Syndrome, you might struggle to internalize your victories and feel uneasy about receiving praise. You might find yourself attributing your successes to others, recalling instances when you collaborated on editing a presentation or coordinating a launch. Thoughts like, "This was truly a team effort, not just me" or "Because I didn't accomplish this entirely on my own, it doesn't really count as an achievement" may cross your mind. It's common to grasp onto any evidence that seems to confirm feelings of unworthiness. However, it's essential to recognize your individual contributions and allow yourself to acknowledge and celebrate your successes.

You might underestimate the value of networking in securing new opportunities and find yourself thinking that any sort of help that you receive through a professional connection somehow diminishes your achievement when dealing with Imposter Syndrome. You may tell yourself, "This success is solely due to my investor's connection," or "Because I wouldn't have made it through the door without my uncle's help, it doesn't really count." It's crucial to recognize that leveraging connections is a valid and common part of professional growth. Your accomplishments, even when facilitated by networking, still reflect your skills and qualifications.

Embracing the role of networking in your success can help shift your perspective and boost your confidence in your abilities.

Struggling with the acceptance of genuine praise can present a considerable challenge. There's a persistent tendency to cast doubt on the authenticity of compliments, often attributing them to mere politeness. You might catch yourself thinking, "They have to say that; it would be impolite not to," or "The only reason he's congratulating me is because he's a nice person, not because I genuinely deserve it." This reluctance to embrace praise can be rooted in a belief that others are merely extending courtesy rather than recognizing the true merit of your accomplishments.

This inclination to downplay positive feedback may hinder your ability to internalize and appreciate your achievements fully. It's important to recognize that compliments are not merely social niceties; more often than not, they reflect genuine appreciation for your skills and contributions. Actively acknowledging and internalizing these positive affirmations can serve as a potent tool in counteracting the effects of Imposter Syndrome. By embracing and valuing positive feedback, you empower yourself to confront self-doubt and build a more resilient and confident mindset.

With Imposter Syndrome, you might find yourself under immense internal pressure to steer clear of failure, fearing exposure as a fake. Paradoxically, as you achieve more success, the pressure intensifies due to heightened responsibility and visibility. Thoughts might race through your mind, like, "I have to give 300% to live up to this," or "I've got to work even harder than everyone else to prevent them from discovering who I really am." This escalating cycle can lead to a sense of urgency and desperation to continually prove yourself, creating a challenging loop of heightened expectations and self-imposed pressure. It's important to recognize this pattern and strive for a more balanced perspective on your achievements to break free from the cycle of frantic self-validation.

Moreover, you might notice yourself using a lot of minimizing language because full confidence feels elusive. You may catch yourself saying or thinking, "I'm not sure if this might work" or "I'm just checking in," employing words like "might," "just," and "kind of " that downplay your contributions. This tendency to minimize your language could stem from a lack of full confidence in your abilities. Being mindful of such language and consciously working to express yourself with more certainty can be a powerful step in overcoming Imposter Syndrome. Embracing assertive language reflects a greater sense of self-assurance and can positively impact how others perceive your confidence and competence.

You might be experiencing the symptoms of Imposter Syndrome without fully recognizing them. Many individuals fail to grasp these signs, choosing to deny or ignore them altogether. However, to conquer the imposter phenomenon, it's crucial to acknowledge that you are struggling with this syndrome. Once you come to this realization, it becomes more feasible to address and apply exercises that assist in navigating through it. The first essential step in overcoming any challenge is acknowledging what you're experiencing and understanding the potential reasons behind it. By recognizing and accepting the presence of Imposter Syndrome, you pave the way for effective strategies to manage and overcome it.

If you're someone who's constantly craving more success, better outcomes, and higher prestige. Despite putting in extensive hard work and achieving ambitious goals, the pursuit of perfection often leaves you feeling unsatisfied. It becomes a relentless cycle where every accomplishment seems overshadowed by the desire for an even higher standard of achievement. Identifying and finding balance in your pursuit of excellence is vital to achieving contentment and recognizing the value in your accomplishments.

You could also be the kind of person who thrives on showcasing their ability to handle an extensive workload in a brief timeframe. You're willing to put in extra hours to secure validation from both colleagues and managers. Your motivation lies in proving that you possess the capability to manage any task thrown your way. However, it's essential to recognize that while demonstrating competence is commendable, finding a sustainable balance between work and well-being is equally important for long-term success and fulfillment.

Your focus is on swiftly and smoothly completing tasks, firmly believing that you got it right on the first try. If you resonate with this imposter - feedback, critique, or the need for rework may feel threatening because, in your perspective, not getting it right initially equals failure. Despite putting minimal effort into your work, you often find success, and this pattern of minimal effort yielding positive results may have been consistent throughout your life. However, it's crucial to recognize that there might come a point where additional effort becomes necessary. Embracing constructive feedback and acknowledging the potential for improvement can contribute to sustained success in the long run.

You may find yourself uninterested in seeking support from others for your work. In fact, you might even harbor resentment toward others. If you identify with this symptom, asking for help is not something you're willing to do, regardless of the situation, as it makes you feel vulnerable and exposes areas where you might lack knowledge or skills. However, it's important to recognize that seeking assistance is not a sign of weakness; rather, it's an opportunity for growth and collaboration that can enhance your overall capabilities. Acknowledging the value of support can contribute positively to your personal and professional development.

You might struggle with realistically assessing your

competence and skills. You could find yourself attributing your success to external factors, criticizing your own performance, and harboring a fear that you won't live up to expectations. In addition, you might notice tendencies to overachieve, sabotaging your success in the process. Self-doubt could be a persistent companion, making it challenging to recognize your achievements genuinely. Setting exceedingly challenging goals may be a pattern for you, and falling short of these objectives might lead to feelings of disappointment.

Imagine Megan, a talented graphic designer who recently landed a job at a prestigious design agency. Despite her impressive portfolio and the successful completion of challenging projects, Megan consistently feels like she doesn't belong among her highly skilled and experienced colleagues.

Whenever her work receives praise, Megan attributes it to luck or assumes her colleagues are just being polite. She often downplays her contributions in team meetings, thinking that others could have done the same, if not better. Even though she meets deadlines and produces high-quality designs, Megan lives in constant fear that her colleagues will discover she's not as talented as they think.

Megan is reluctant to seek feedback or ask for help, fearing that doing so would expose her lack of expertise. She overworks herself, putting in long hours to prove her worth. Despite external validation and success in her projects, Megan remains convinced that she's just "faking it" and that, eventually, everyone will realize she's not as competent as they believe.

The above scenario exemplifies the classic traits of Imposter Syndrome, where an individual with significant accomplishments and capabilities doubts their own abilities, feels like a fraud, and fears being exposed as incompetent despite evidence to the contrary.

Recognizing these patterns is the first step toward overcoming

Imposter Syndrome. It's essential to cultivate a more balanced perspective on your abilities and accomplishments, allowing for a healthier and more realistic assessment of your skills.

However, if you're navigating the path to identify and overcome your unique Imposter Syndrome patterns, here are some steps that could help you.

You should recognize that success is a subjective concept, varying from person to person. Acknowledge that what one person deems successful might differ from another. It's essential to embrace your achievements, whether they're monumental or small, without subjecting yourself to harsh self-judgment. Remember, your journey is unique, and comparing yourself to others can be counterproductive. Celebrate your individual successes and the personal growth they represent. By appreciating your distinctive path, you'll find greater satisfaction and confidence in your accomplishments. Take pride in your progress, and don't be too hard on yourself. Each step forward is a testament to your capabilities and resilience.

Begin with establishing boundaries around systems or individuals that may be hindering your personal wellness and growth. Identify environments or relationships contributing to feelings of inadequacy and set clear limits to safeguard your well-being. Remember, prioritizing spaces that nurture your personal growth and positive self-perception is crucial. Surround yourself with supportive people and environments that empower you rather than drain your energy. Recognize that it's okay to distance yourself from negativity and prioritize your mental and emotional health. By creating these boundaries, you ensure a more conducive and uplifting space for your personal development.

Take ownership of your objective successes. Celebrate your accomplishments, attributing them to your skills and hard work. Don't sell yourself short by attributing achievements solely to external factors. It's important to acknowledge your competence and expertise, recognizing that your efforts and abilities contribute significantly to your successes. Embrace the recognition of your skills and the value you bring to the table. By internalizing your achievements, you build a stronger sense of confidence and empower yourself to pursue even greater goals. Remember, your capabilities play a key role in your success, so give yourself the credit you deserve.

Incorporate consistent self-care check-ins into your routine. Regularly assess your mental and emotional well-being to ensure a healthy balance in your life. Identify activities that not only bring you joy and relaxation but also align with your personal preferences. Make these activities a regular part of your routine, as they play a fundamental role in maintaining a balanced and healthy lifestyle. Remember to prioritize your well-being, and don't hesitate to adjust your self-care practices based on your evolving needs. Establishing these regular check-ins and nurturing activities will contribute to your overall happiness and resilience in the face of life's challenges.

Consider reaching out to a therapist. Seeking guidance from a professional tailored to your experience with Imposter Syndrome can be transformative. Engage in open conversations with a therapist to create a supportive space for developing effective coping strategies and cultivating a mindset conducive to well-being. Remember, seeking support is a strength, and acknowledging the need for assistance is a commendable step in your journey toward self-discovery. Your mental and emotional well-being is a valuable investment in your overall happiness, and a therapist can provide valuable insights to help you navigate the challenges posed by Imposter Syndrome. Don't hesitate to take this proactive step toward a healthier and more confident version of yourself.

These insights are essential for boosting self-confidence and finding fulfillment, both professionally and personally. Recognizing and dealing with these patterns marks a substantial step toward embracing your capabilities and cultivating a more balanced and positive mindset.

Chapter 3
Impact of Imposter Syndrome on Career

Although Imposter Syndrome can affect individuals in all areas of life, it's particularly common in high-achieving persons at work. As you explore the impact of Imposter Syndrome on careers, you'll notice its widespread presence in workplaces. Once you recognize it in yourself, you'll realize the undeniable effect it has on your career. This awareness helps you understand how it influences your confidence, career choices, and job satisfaction. Acknowledging Imposter Syndrome is the first step to navigating its impact on your professional life and taking proactive measures to address it.

Let's talk about all the ways through which Imposter Syndrome could be making an entrance into your professional lives. For instance, you could be the one putting in all the hard work required, diligently achieving each goal on time. However, despite your progress, there's a lingering feeling that your success holds no real value. It's as if the effort you invest somehow doesn't measure up to the accomplishments you attain. This disconnects between your achievements and the recognition of their significance contributes to a sense of undervaluation, casting a shadow on your otherwise commendable efforts.

Most days, you don't even have the slightest realization of how you've just numbed yourself to go about with your life, because it's pretty normalized in today's hustle culture to wear yourself out during your peak years of life. You are constantly told and preached about how these years, which are meant to be your most productive and energetic ones, are the ones in which you need to hustle to your maximum capacity so that you can lay back and relax during your mid-forties and onwards. However, these very energetic years are also the ones in which you're supposed to live life a little. Unfortunately, with all the chaos and competition, you forget to breathe, to live, and to laugh to your heart's content.

Relentlessly pushing yourself to exhibit your maximum potential in every domain and niche of your career, testing your limits and capacities, you end up exhausting yourself to the core. Whether it's arriving early or staying late every day, dedicating your time off to work, or attending every optional meeting, you're putting in extraordinary effort. This ruthless commitment to your work is admirable, but it's crucial to recognize the potential toll it can take on your well-being. Balancing dedication with self-care is essential to ensure sustained productivity and overall personal health.

You even beat yourself up for even the smallest mistakes. To you, nothing less than perfection is acceptable. Even though you might be lenient with others, you find it challenging to "let the little things go" when it comes to yourself. This self-imposed standard can lead to unnecessary stress and a constant feeling of falling short of your own expectations. It's important to recognize that everyone makes mistakes, and allowing yourself some grace can contribute to a healthier and more balanced mindset.

You might be someone who constantly perceives yourself as unworthy of your position. There's a lingering fear that you might be "found out" by your boss or co-workers, and you carry the persistent sense that you're fooling people by merely appearing to do a good job. This perception of inadequacy can create unnecessary anxiety, affecting your confidence in the workplace. It's essential to recognize that your accomplishments are valid and the expertise you bring to your role is genuinely valuable. While you feel like a fraud, everyone else around you appear competent and successful in comparison. You're convinced your colleagues have it all together. The belief that you're the only one struggling with imposter feelings intensifies, contributing to a sense of isolation. It's crucial to recognize that many individuals, even those who seem confident, may deal with similar doubts. Remember, appearances can be deceiving, and you're not alone in facing the complexities of competence and success in the workplace.

Do you find it challenging to accept praise or compliments? Despite everyone else saying you're doing great, you never think your work is good enough. Every instance of receiving praise or promotion is overshadowed by your inner critic speaking so loudly that the accomplishments fail to register. This self-critical perspective diminishes the joy and satisfaction that should accompany your successes. It's essential to quiet that inner voice, acknowledge your achievements, and appreciate the recognition you receive for your hard work and accomplishments. Embracing positive feedback can be a powerful tool in battling the impact of Imposter Syndrome.

You've started neglecting self-care. When you're too busy with work or drained from your long days, you might not take the time you need to recharge. This neglect of self-care is a common symptom of burnout, which often accompanies imposter syndrome. It's crucial to recognize the interconnection of your well-being and professional challenges. Prioritizing self-care can be a transformative step in managing the pressures of work and maintaining a healthy balance between your personal and professional life. Remember, taking care of yourself is not a luxury but a necessity for sustained success and fulfillment.

Additionally, you might find yourself believing that your job or career status defines who you are. Instead of bringing your authentic self to your job, it seems as though your job brings you closer to understanding yourself. It's essential to recognize that your identity extends beyond your professional role, and embracing your unique qualities can contribute significantly to your overall fulfillment and personal growth.

When such self-doubting feelings start infiltrating your daily work experiences, they not only cast a shadow on your mood but also create barriers between you and success. It's necessary to acknowledge and address these moments of uncertainty, as overcoming them can pave the way for a more positive and productive journey toward achieving your goals. Embrace your strengths, confront doubts head-on, and watch how your path to success becomes clearer and more fulfilling.

But here's the thing: you don't have to let Imposter Syndrome win. There are several effective ways for you to fight it. It is a fact that you are not the only one feeling this way; many successful individuals have faced similar doubts. Recognize your achievements and give yourself credit for your hard work. Remember that everyone makes mistakes and experiences setbacks - it's a normal part of the learning process. Surround yourself with a support system of friends, mentors, or colleagues who can offer encouragement and perspective. Challenge negative thoughts by focusing on your strengths and accomplishments. Set realistic goals and celebrate your progress along the way. By taking these steps, you can reclaim your confidence and overcome Imposter Syndrome.

Start by learning to focus on your strengths as much as you do on your weaknesses. Surely, there are areas where you can grow, but there's a lot where you're already doing many things right. Take the time to pinpoint those natural strengths; they are the qualities that make you stand out and excel. Accept the uniqueness of your skills and talents. Don't forget to celebrate your achievements - both big and small. By acknowledging what you're already doing well, you'll build a foundation of confidence that will drive you forward in your journey of personal and professional growth.

For instance, let's say you find yourself uneasy with networking events and face-to-face interactions, but you thrive in expressing ideas through visual means. Instead of solely concentrating on overcoming social discomfort, invest more time practicing your skills in graphic design or creating visually compelling presentations. This shift not only allows you to excel in an area where you feel more comfortable but can also pave the way for exciting opportunities that align with your genuine interests and strengths. Stop neglecting the areas you already shine in - and see how you can get even better at what you already rock at.

It would be best if you learn to forgive yourself for your mistakes and understand that they don't only happen to you. Instead of criticizing yourself for "yet another mistake" or thinking, "I always make mistakes at work," learn to acknowledge that errors are a universal part of everyone's life. The next time you make a mistake - let's say you accidentally send an email before finishing it or miss a deadline, remind yourself: You are not the mistake, and the mistake does not define you or your career.

Also, remember that your colleagues and supervisors have made mistakes before, just like you! Whether you can see these mistakes or not, understand that everyone around you is just as fallible as you are. It's easy to assume that others have it all together, but the truth is they've faced their share of challenges and slip-ups. Don't hesitate to share your experiences with colleagues; it fosters a culture of openness and understanding. By recognizing that everyone is on their own journey of learning and growth, you'll feel more connected and supported in your professional environment. Accept the lesson they offer and use it to become even more skilled and resilient in your professional journey. It's not about avoiding mistakes but about learning from them and moving forward together.

Know that your response to a mistake matters more than the mistake itself. Always keep in mind the saying, "It is not what happens to you, but how you react to it that matters." When faced with a misstep, focus on your reaction and the steps you take to address and learn from it. Instead of focusing on the error, channel your energy into finding constructive solutions and implementing positive changes. Realize that setbacks are opportunities for personal and professional development. By cultivating a resilient and proactive mindset, you'll not only navigate challenges more effectively but also demonstrate to yourself and others the strength of your character in the face of adversity.

Think of it this way: Once a mistake is made, you can't change it. However, the next move is always within your control. Take charge by being honest and opening up about the mistake immediately. Reflect on where you went wrong and the events that led to the mistake. Consider how you can resolve the situation, both in the present and in the future, to prevent further incidents.

Use the experience as a valuable lesson to enhance your decision-making skills. Seek feedback from others to gain different perspectives and insights. Embrace the opportunity for growth and demonstrate your commitment to continuous improvement. Remember, it's not about avoiding mistakes altogether but about responding with resilience, accountability, and a positive mindset. Taking ownership of your actions and learning from blunders is a powerful way to build trust and genuineness in both your career and personal life.

The aim should be to strive for the best and not for perfection. When you pressure yourself to be perfect, you may feel anxious and end up making more mistakes. It's paradoxical, but accepting the fact that mistakes happen can actually help you be more relaxed and make fewer of them. Understand that expecting perfection is unrealistic and doesn't give you the flexibility to develop course-correcting skills for when mistakes do occur. Give yourself the freedom to learn and grow from your experiences. Set realistic standards that allow room for improvement without the burden of unattainable perfection.

Make room for the process of continual improvement, and view mistakes as valuable opportunities to refine your skills. This mindset not only reduces stress but also fosters resilience and adaptability. Remember, the pursuit of your best self involves progress, not perfection. Celebrate your achievements, no matter how small, and keep challenging yourself to reach new heights, knowing that each step forward is a significant accomplishment.

Imagine you have a fantastic idea at work, one that could truly make a difference. However, Imposter Syndrome creeps in, making you doubt your abilities and causing you to hesitate. In the end, you decide not to share your idea in a meeting. The consequence? The project moves forward without your valuable input, and the missed opportunity could have been a turning point for your career. Likewise, consider a scenario where a job opening aligns perfectly with your skills and passions, but Imposter Syndrome convinces you that you're not qualified. You decide not to apply, letting the opportunity slip away. In the meantime, someone else who may have similar skills, but a more confident approach lands the position, leaving you to wonder about the potential growth and fulfillment you could have experienced.

In personal relationships, Imposter Syndrome might lead you to downplay your achievements or hesitate to pursue new connections. This reluctance to share your true self can hold back the depth and authenticity of your relationships, both personally and professionally. People around you may not fully appreciate your talents and capabilities, and you might miss out on collaborations, mentorships, or friendships that could have enriched your life.

Over time, the toll of unaddressed Imposter Syndrome can accumulate. It may lead to a chronic sense of dissatisfaction as you consistently underestimate your worth and capabilities. This could result in affecting your mental health, leading to stress, anxiety, and a diminished sense of self-esteem. Ultimately, not addressing Imposter Syndrome or not acknowledging it as a real issue can hinder your overall well-being, limit your professional growth, and prevent you from realizing your full potential. It is perfectly alright if you're dealing with Imposter Syndrome but denying it and not taking action could be detrimental to your mental health. Remember, it's not just about professional success; it's about unlocking a more fulfilling and balanced life for yourself. Your mental well-being is important because when it's good, everything else seems to flourish too.

Creating boundaries is healthy; it is a sign of self-respect and a mandatory step in maintaining a healthy balance in your life. It's okay for you to say no. You're only human, and you can't do everything at once or be perfect at everything you do - perfection is unrealistic and can lead to unnecessary stress. Making mistakes is a human tendency; stumbling and falling are alright - as long as you know how to get back on your feet. Learning comes with making mistakes, as they contribute to your growth and resilience. You're not obligated to live up to everyone's expectations. Prioritize self-care; you must focus on yourself and your health and never hesitate to communicate your needs to others. Give yourself the space to be truly human. By valuing yourself and establishing healthy boundaries, you create an environment that supports your overall well-being and allows you to thrive authentically.

Chapter 4
Imposter Syndrome in Leadership

In leadership, Imposter Syndrome might be affecting you if you notice behaviors like perfectionism and overworking. These feelings can make you believe you're not qualified for your position, even when you are. It's a common phenomenon that can impact professionals at every career level and in various organizations and industries. While having high standards and being detail-oriented is commendable, it's essential to admit that no one benefits when team members burn out.

The most effective leaders understand that good mental and physical health is key to performance, and they empower their teams to tend to their well-being, too. Employees need to feel that they are valued as whole people with unique talents and goals. This is why empathy is a prime attribute of successful leaders. Teams thrive when individuals feel understood, validated, and connected to one another. This Whole Person perspective has been shown to drive innovation, employee engagement, and business results, but also the psychological resources that sustain high-performing leaders over time.

Step away from the all-work-no-play mindset by developing effective stress management and self-compassion in your leadership approach. Rather than scheduling back-to-back meetings, intentionally structure your calendar to include breaks, allowing yourself the time to decompress and recharge. Prioritize taking vacations, recognizing the value of stepping back to rejuvenate your mind and spirit. It's essential to acknowledge that you can't handle everything, and that's not only acceptable but a wise recognition of your human limitations. Embrace the power of delegation, moving away from the image of a tough individualist who tackles everything alone. Empower your team by distributing responsibilities according to strengths and expertise, fostering a collaborative and supportive work culture.

Consider setting the tone for work-life balance by encouraging your team to take breaks, prioritize self-care, and utilize their vacation time. As a leader, your actions speak louder than words, and by demonstrating the importance of a balanced approach, you create an environment where your team feels empowered to do the same. Effective leadership goes beyond productivity metrics; it involves nurturing the well-being of both yourself and your team. By weaving stress management, self-compassion, and a collaborative mindset into your leadership style, you contribute to a workplace that values both professional excellence and the health and happiness of its members.

Instead of praising your team member's intelligence or talent, focus on acknowledging the effort they put into the task. Psychological research suggests that praising effort, like saying, "You worked really hard on this," is the most effective way to foster a strong sense of self-esteem and prevent Imposter Syndrome.

Celebrate incremental progress not only to keep your morale high but also to help you internalize success. Consider creating a brag file - a document where you log your wins at work, regardless of size. This practice allows you to look back on your accomplishments with a healthy sense of pride, preventing you from dismissing them as mere luck or connections. It can even prove handy during performance reviews, helping you prepare to take ownership of your responsibilities. Acknowledging your efforts and documenting your achievements builds a positive mindset, reducing the likelihood of feeling like an imposter. By focusing on the processes and progress, you create a foundation of confidence that strengthens your self-esteem and fosters a healthier perspective on your professional accomplishments.

Utilize Self-Assessment and 360-degree Feedback tools to uncover opportunities for your learning and development in a growth-oriented way. Empower your team by leveraging feedback to ensure a clear understanding of expectations, ultimately reducing unnecessary self-doubt among individual contributors.

As you engage with tools, actively seek out opportunities for learning and skill development. These tools serve as valuable resources for your growth-oriented approach, helping you identify areas where you can expand your expertise and capabilities. Embrace the feedback loop, as it not only enhances your understanding of expectations but also fosters a collaborative environment where continuous improvement is encouraged.

Support your team by encouraging each member to take an inventory of their strengths, possibly with the guidance of a coach (a leader can always teach their juniors). A skilled coach can assist you in fully leveraging your strengths, bringing out unique attributes that make you shine in your work. Work closely with the coach to identify these strengths and develop consistent actions and habits that propel you toward success at your full potential. When you identify opportunities for personal development, it's natural to experience moments of self-doubt. Understand that taking on a challenge or embracing a new responsibility can create a sense of vulnerability for you.

In these situations, it's important to encourage yourself and those around you to approach the practice with a healthy dose of self-compassion. Know that growth involves stepping into the unknown, and by embracing it with kindness toward yourself, you pave the way for meaningful development and success. Approaching your development as a series of low-stakes experiments can also be beneficial. Confidence is a skill that can be learned. Infusing a sense of playfulness into the process not only makes it more enjoyable but also cultivates resilience. This way, when setbacks inevitably occur, you and everyone involved can bounce back with greater ease.

To cultivate an environment for open discussions where you and your team can feel at ease, expressing themselves without the fear of being perceived as incompetent. It's essential to establish a space for candid conversations. Begin by setting communication ground rules made to foster inclusion:

1. **Ensure No Interruptions:** Encourage everyone, including yourself, to actively listen without interrupting. This creates a respectful atmosphere where each person's thoughts can be fully expressed.

2. **Provide Equal Speaking Time:** Allocate equal time for each team member to share their perspectives. This ensures that everyone has an opportunity to contribute to the conversation and helps in building an inclusive conversation.

3. **Acknowledge Mistakes, Wins, and Opportunities:** Emphasize the importance of acknowledging not only mistakes but also celebrating wins and recognizing opportunities for development. This balanced approach promotes a positive and constructive communication culture.

4. **Encourage Constructive Feedback:** Foster an environment where constructive feedback is welcomed. This helps individuals grow, learn from each other, and contribute to the continuous improvement of the team.

5. **Express Gratitude:** Encourage expressing gratitude and appreciation for the efforts and contributions of team members. This positivity reinforces a supportive atmosphere within the team.

By implementing these communication ground rules, you

create a space that values everyone's input and promotes a sense of belonging. This sets the foundation for candid conversations, where ideas flow freely, and each team member feels empowered to speak up without hesitation.

On your professional journey, the support of a leader can be beneficial for everyone, but it holds particular significance for underrepresented groups. Engaging in mentoring, seeking sponsorships, and participating in diversity training can effectively lessen the adverse impacts of unconscious bias and the feeling of being an outsider. By actively pursuing these opportunities, you can work to alleviate the effects of Imposter Syndrome on your self-confidence. Taking charge to lead from a place of vulnerability and modeling resilience becomes necessary in this effort, showcasing that overcoming challenges is not only possible but also an integral part of growth and success. However, your journey is unique, and seeking support and guidance can be a powerful step toward realizing your full potential and navigating the professional landscape with confidence and authenticity.

Research indicates that sensitive individuals, are often highly attuned to their thoughts, feelings, and the reactions of others. As a Sensitive Striver, you might find yourself struggling with Imposter Syndrome - feeling like a fake or fraud at work - more than most. The good news is there's a way out for you. Take the initiative to learn how to remain calm and composed under pressure instead of freezing. Replace sabotaging thoughts with an empowering inner dialogue. Reimagine your goal-setting approach to foster more self-trust and momentum. Liberate yourself from draining comparisons that divert your focus and embrace a mindset that celebrates your unique strengths and contributions. Keep in mind that overcoming Imposter Syndrome is a journey. Actively working on these aspects can help build a sense of self-assurance and belief in your professional pursuits.

Nevertheless, Imposter Syndrome can show up in different ways, and you might be familiar with one or more types at the same time. Here are some common ones you might identify with:

1. **The Perfectionist**: You might identify this type of imposter in yourself - you feel a constant need to excel and attain perfection in every task. Setting exceedingly high standards, you often fear being revealed as inadequate, especially when facing even minor mistakes. It's important to understand that many individuals share this experience, and overcoming it involves recognizing the value of progress over perfection. Embrace the journey of learning and growth, admitting that mistakes are a natural part of the process and not a reflection of your overall competence. Seek support and celebrate your achievements, fostering a mindset that values effort and improvement rather than an unattainable standard of flawlessness.

2. **The Expert**: This is a type of Imposter Syndrome, where you believe you must know everything before taking on a task or accepting recognition for your work. Feeling the need to be an expert in all areas and having a fear of being perceived as incompetent or lacking knowledge. It's crucial to recognize that no one knows everything, and seeking help or learning along the way is a sign of strength, not weakness. Adopt a mindset that values continuous learning and acknowledges that expertise is a journey, not a fixed destination. Remember, it's okay to grow and expand your knowledge, and doing so contributes to your professional development.

3. **The Natural Genius**: You might find that you relate to this type of Imposter Syndrome, where you believe you should effortlessly excel in all areas without much effort or struggle. Feeling ineffective and experiencing

self-doubt can be common when you encounter challenges or need to put in extra effort to succeed. It's helpful to understand that everyone faces obstacles, and putting in effort is a natural part of growth and achievement. Hold on to the learning process and understand that your worth is not solely determined by how easily things come to you. Celebrate your efforts and progress, acknowledging that challenges are opportunities for development and not reflections of your inherent abilities.

4. **The Soloist**: You might recognize this tendency in yourself, where you feel the need to accomplish tasks on your own as a Soloist. There might be hesitancy to ask for help or support, driven by a fear that seeking assistance could reveal perceived incompetence or dependence on others. It's essential to understand that asking for help is a strength, not a weakness. Involving collaboration in your work and recognizing that seeking support doesn't diminish your abilities; rather, it fosters a collective effort toward success. By accepting that everyone benefits from collaboration, you can build a stronger foundation for personal and professional growth.

5. **The Superhero**: You might notice this type of Imposter Syndrome in yourself - you tend to take on excessive workloads and responsibilities, going above and beyond what is expected of you. There might be a fear of disappointing others, and you often feel the need to prove your worth through constant overachievement. It's important to recognize that your accomplishments do not solely define your value, and it's okay to set boundaries. A balanced approach that values your well-being alongside your professional contributions is needed. Seek validation in your achievements but also in your ability to maintain a healthy work-life balance. Remember, your worth goes

beyond the quantity of tasks you undertake, and finding a sustainable pace is essential for long-term success and fulfillment.

6. **The Outsider**: The kind of Imposter Syndrome where you feel like you don't belong or that you are different from your colleagues or peers. There could be a tendency to attribute your achievements to external factors like luck or being in the right place at the right time rather than recognizing your own capabilities. It would help if you accepted the fact that you are not alone in feeling this way, and many individuals share similar experiences. Embrace the idea that your achievements are a result of your skills and efforts, and you deserve the success you've achieved. Work on developing a positive self-image and focus on your unique strengths that contribute to the collective success of your team or peers. Remember, you belong, and your contributions are valuable.

It's important for you to note that these types are not mutually exclusive, and you might find yourself experiencing a combination of different Imposter Syndrome types. Recognizing and understanding these patterns can be helpful for both individuals and organizations to address and provide support for those dealing with Imposter Syndrome. By accepting the complexity of these experiences, you can work towards cultivating a supportive environment that encourages authenticity, self-awareness, and a positive mindset. You're not alone, and there are strategies and resources available to help you navigate and overcome Imposter Syndrome.

Leading can be challenging, balancing the responsibility of not overwhelming your team while ensuring the work gets done. Patience is crucial in dealing with teammates of varying personalities, as there are times when you teach and other times when you learn from them. It's common to question your leadership skills, feeling the Imposter Syndrome creeping in, but it's important to stay composed and acknowledge that you're doing your best.

Chapter 5
Overcoming Imposter Syndrome

In the earlier chapters, we explored the complex concept of imposter syndrome, breaking down its definition and offering insights into identifying its presence in personal and professional aspects. We also dived into the extensive impact that imposter syndrome can have on one's career. As we move forward, our exploration continues with a focus on practical strategies. We aim to not only overcome imposter syndrome but also to manage this phenomenon effectively, empowering ourselves to skillfully navigate the challenges it presents.

In flexible working environments, several factors can contribute to the development of imposter syndrome. Understanding these influences is important for effectively addressing and overcoming this phenomenon. We will discuss some main factors and corresponding strategies to help you overcome them. Realizing the importance of valuing your employees is necessary.

Suppose you sense that you need more acknowledgment. In that case, it's often linked to a lack of clarity in your job expectations, feedback on your performance, the recognition you receive, and the support for your professional growth. Effective communication becomes pivotal in addressing these concerns. Make sure you understand your company's vision and goals and how your efforts tie into the larger picture. By fostering clear communication channels, you not only enhance your sense of value but also contribute more meaningfully to the overarching objectives of the organization. Your role is integral, and your contributions matter in the broader context of the company's success.

If you find yourself struggling with Imposter Syndrome in your flexible work setup, take a moment to evaluate your perception of your organization's vision and goals. Ensure that your leader and key stakeholders share the same understanding. Additionally, it's crucial to evaluate whether your colleagues recognize the value you bring and can clearly see how your efforts contribute to the company's overarching objectives. By engaging in this self-reflection and open communication, you can reinforce your confidence and strengthen the connection between your work and the broader goals of the organization. Aligning your understanding with that of your leaders and peers is key to overcoming Imposter Syndrome and thriving in your flexible work environment.

Believing in your own values and abilities creates a healthy mindset and helps in overcoming the Imposter Syndrome. Make it a habit to consistently communicate your accomplishments and actively seek feedback. This not only helps those around you acknowledge your worth but also serves to boost your confidence in your capacity to contribute effectively within a flexible working environment. By sharing your successes and inviting constructive input, you not only enhance your own perception of your capabilities but also foster a positive and collaborative work environment. Remember, your unique skills are valuable, and regularly showcasing them contributes to a more supportive and appreciative professional atmosphere.

However, suppose you ever find yourself in a situation where you're not receiving equal treatment or fair pay. In such circumstances, it's crucial to begin by evaluating whether you have advocated for yourself by expressing your worth. Once you've taken this step and encountered resistance, it becomes necessary to delve deeper into the root cause of the issue. Investigating the factors at play can help identify any disparities and pave the way for informed actions to address the situation appropriately.

Promoting fair treatment and compensation is an essential

aspect of ensuring a just and equitable professional environment. It's vital to explore whether the issue stems from a lack of communication and understanding or if it's rooted in a toxic workplace culture that undervalues its employees. Take a moment to reflect on whether educating and engaging in an open dialogue with your employer could bridge the gap. Sometimes, seeking clarity through communication is essential. However, if your intuition signals that something isn't right, trust your instincts and take the initiative to gather the necessary facts. Understanding the dynamics at play empowers you to make informed decisions about how to address the situation and advocate for your rights in the workplace. Your well-being and fair treatment are the two things that matter the most.

Acknowledge your value and be prepared to speak up, whether negotiating for fair compensation or seeking a supportive work environment. Recognizing and communicating your worth not only helps your professional development but also encourages a workplace that values your contributions. Have the confidence to advocate for what you deserve, paving the way for a more satisfying and fair professional journey. Asserting your worth is a significant step in creating a positive and respectful work environment.

In considering whether flexible working should impact your career progression, ideally, in a forward-thinking organization, your answer should be a resounding "No." However, in certain workplaces, it might, unless you proactively take crucial steps to safeguard your professional growth and dig into your own emotional intelligence. By being proactive and staying attuned to your emotional intelligence, you can navigate the nuances of flexible work arrangements and ensure that they do not hinder your career advancement.

When you're joining an organization, it's essential to thoroughly research and understand their stance on flexible working and confirm they offer progression opportunities for those who choose this path. Don't hesitate to inquire about these opportunities, and if they seem nonexistent, consider it a red flag. As a flexible worker, make sure to share your motivations and aspirations with your employer, emphasizing the benefits of supporting your growth in a non-traditional work arrangement. Incorporate your flexible working goals into every personal development plan and communicate them with your team. It's important for you to make your employer recognize the value of accommodating flexible workers; otherwise, there's a risk of losing exceptional talent to more forward-thinking competitors. Taking an active role in shaping your professional journey within the organization ensures that your flexible work arrangement aligns with your career goals and contributes positively to the overall success of the team.

As a flexible worker, you might encounter another challenge closely tied to the value discussion earlier - visibility within the organization. Working remotely, on compressed hours, or following different patterns than your colleagues can sometimes leave you feeling less seen. It's important for you to actively address this by finding opportunities to showcase your contributions. Consider scheduling regular check-ins with your team, participating in virtual meetings, and proactively sharing your accomplishments. By actively seeking visibility, you ensure that your valuable contributions are acknowledged and appreciated, even in a non-traditional work setting. Remember, taking these steps enhances your professional presence and strengthens your connection with your colleagues and the organization as a whole. In your flexible work scenario, feelings of Imposter Syndrome may manifest in various ways. You might find yourself thinking that bosses and colleagues are less aware of your contributions to the company. There could be concerns that you're perceived as less committed because you're not physically present in the office from 9 to 5. You need to recognize these potential challenges and actively address them. Seek opportunities to communicate your achievements and highlight your commitment to your work, regardless of the physical workspace. By taking these steps, you can combat feelings of being undervalued and ensure that your impact on the organization is acknowledged and appreciated. Your contributions are valuable, and actively managing your visibility is key to overcoming Imposter Syndrome in a flexible work environment.

Nevertheless, you must remember that you bring unique value to an organization, regardless of your working pattern. Your role is enriched by the wealth of experience, knowledge, and passion you contribute, and your commitment is no less significant than someone adhering to a more traditional work style. Embrace the understanding that your individuality and the distinctive perspectives you bring are assets that contribute to the overall success of the organization. Don't underestimate the impact of your contributions, and actively communicate your value within the context of your flexible work arrangement. By recognizing and appreciating your worth, you contribute to a workplace culture that values diversity and acknowledges the varied strengths each team member brings to the table.

However, it's easy to find yourself wondering about strategies to overcome Imposter Syndrome. Begin with assessing whether your thoughts and feelings are grounded in reality or personal insecurities - it's a helpful first step. Engage in open discussions with your leaders to express your feelings and contribute to shaping a more supportive working environment. This may involve suggesting solutions, such as strategies to enhance visibility in team meetings or proposing more regular touchpoints with management. By actively participating in these conversations, you not only address Imposter Syndrome but also play a role in fostering a work environment that aligns with your needs and contributes to your professional growth. Your insights and contributions are valuable, and taking active steps can make a meaningful difference in overcoming Imposter Syndrome in a flexible work setting.

To overcome Imposter Syndrome in this scenario, consider implementing the following strategies.

Reality Check: When dealing with Imposter Syndrome, pause to check if your thoughts are based on reality or insecurities. Challenge negative self-perceptions by focusing on evidence of your skills and achievements. Recall specific instances of competence and positive feedback to boost confidence. Regularly acknowledge your strengths, creating a positive self-perception. Consistently reinforcing your abilities helps combat Imposter Syndrome and fosters a mindset reflecting your true value.

Open Discussions: Initiate open conversations with your leaders to address Imposter Syndrome. Share your feelings and concerns, and work together to create a more supportive and inclusive flexible work environment. Discuss strategies like regular check-ins to validate your contributions and emphasize the importance of open communication. Actively engaging with your leaders contributes to a positive work environment that recognizes the challenges of flexible work arrangements. Your voice can drive positive change in your professional journey.

Suggest Solutions: When engaging in discussions, propose practical solutions to enhance your experience. Consider strategies like increasing your visibility in team meetings through regular updates on your contributions. You might also advocate for more frequent touchpoints with management to ensure your efforts are recognized and valued. By actively participating in these conversations, you not only address specific challenges but also contribute to a work environment that aligns better with your needs and aspirations. Your input is valuable, and suggesting these solutions demonstrates your commitment to a more supportive and inclusive professional setting.

Seek Feedback: Proactively ask for feedback on your performance. Understanding how others see your contributions provides reassurance and helps counter feelings of inadequacy. Talk with colleagues and supervisors to gain insights into your work's impact. Consider having regular feedback sessions or seeking input on specific projects. Actively seeking feedback enhances self-awareness and shows your commitment to continuous improvement. Remember, feedback is a valuable tool for personal and professional growth, aiding in your development and success in your role.

Self-Affirmation: In cultivating a positive mindset, practice self-affirmation by acknowledging your accomplishments and reminding yourself of the unique value you bring to the organization. Take a positive step by creating a list of your strengths and make it a habit to revisit and reflect on it regularly. When self-doubt creeps in, use this list as a powerful tool to reinforce your confidence. Celebrate both small and significant achievements, recognizing your contributions to the team. By consistently affirming your worth, you build a strong foundation for self-assurance and resilience - essential attributes in navigating the challenges of the workplace. Embracing your strengths contributes not only to your personal well-being but also to the positive dynamics of the organization.

Mentorship and Support: In navigating challenges, seek mentorship or support from colleagues who can offer valuable guidance and perspective. Engage with individuals who have shared experiences to normalize feelings of self-doubt and imposterism. Open conversations with your colleagues about their own professional journeys and the strategies they've employed to overcome similar challenges. By seeking mentorship and sharing experiences, you gain valuable insights and foster a sense of friendship and mutual support within the workplace. Connecting with others who understand your experiences can be a powerful source of encouragement and empowerment in your career journey.

Professional Development Plans: Include your flexible working goals in your career plans. Clearly state your career aspirations and talk with your team to make sure they align with the organization's objectives. Share how flexible work can help your professional growth and the team's success. Keep communication open to discuss any adjustments or support needed. Actively involving your team creates a collaborative environment supporting diverse career paths. Remember, clear communication ensures your goals align with both personal ambitions and the organization's mission.

Networking Opportunities: Get involved in networking opportunities within your organization. Build connections with colleagues to boost your visibility and create a strong support system for handling challenges. Attend team events, virtual meet-ups, and professional gatherings to expand your network. Connecting with colleagues beyond daily tasks can lead to valuable collaborations and opportunities for sharing insights. Building these connections contributes to a more inclusive work environment and positions you for various opportunities within the organization. Keep in mind that networking is a dynamic tool for professional growth, playing a significant role in your career journey.

Celebrate Achievements: Celebrate your achievements, no matter how big or small. Take the time to recognize and acknowledge your successes, reinforcing a positive self-image. Share your accomplishments with colleagues and seek credit for your contributions. Embrace a practical approach by setting aside moments to reflect on your achievements regularly. Consider keeping a success journal to document your progress and revisit it to appreciate your growth. By actively celebrating your successes, you not only boost your confidence but also create a mindset that focuses on continual self-improvement. Acknowledging your achievements is a powerful motivator in cultivating a positive and resilient professional outlook.

Continuous Learning: Adopt a mindset of continuous learning. Stay updated on industry trends and invest in your professional development to boost confidence in your skills. Look out for learning opportunities, whether through online courses, workshops, or networking events. Engage with industry literature and publications to stay informed about the latest developments. Consider joining professional associations or groups to connect with peers and gain diverse insights. By consistently investing in your learning journey, you not only enhance your expertise but also position yourself as an active contributor in your field. Staying curious and committed to ongoing learning is a key driver of professional growth and success.

By using these strategies, you can actively address Imposter Syndrome, developing a positive mindset that supports your growth. Consistently engage with these steps to build resilience and self-confidence over time. Understand that overcoming Imposter Syndrome is an ongoing process, and your efforts significantly contribute to your personal and professional development. Embrace the journey, recognizing that each step is meaningful toward building a more confident version of yourself. Your commitment to these practices benefits you and positively impacts the work environment around you. Keep in mind that small, consistent actions lead to lasting change.

Chapter 6
Building Resilience

You have the power to use resilience as a strong antidote for Imposter Syndrome. This ability helps you overcome challenges, bounce back from setbacks, and foster a positive mindset. When you tap into your resilience, you not only conquer obstacles but also build a mindset that strengthens your abilities and pushes back against the doubts linked to Imposter Syndrome.

In the face of challenges, you can view failures as stepping stones to growth. Each setback becomes an invaluable learning opportunity, allowing you to dismiss feelings of inadequacy and instead recognize the potential for improvement. Your resilience encourages you to adapt to change gracefully, understanding that uncertainties are a natural part of life's journey.

Building self-confidence involves developing trust in your abilities. Resilience helps you embrace continuous improvement, fostering a growth mindset that counters the fixed mindset linked to imposter syndrome. Setting realistic goals becomes a crucial strategy, enabling you to experience success and recognize your progress along the way. Seeking support from others is a strength, not a weakness. Connecting with mentors, friends, or colleagues offers diverse perspectives and valuable feedback, reminding you that you're not alone in facing challenges. Your resilience helps you navigate difficulties and celebrate even small successes, encouraging a positive self-image and reducing the impact of imposter syndrome.

Having a resilient workforce brings numerous benefits, making you and your colleagues more motivated, better at handling change, and less prone to burnout. The connection between resilience and workplace well-being is significant, contributing to improved mental health among employees like yourself. This connection translates into fewer instances of absenteeism and presenteeism, enhancing overall workplace performance. As you and your team build resilience, the positive effects flow through the organization, creating a work environment where adaptability, motivation, and well-being unite for sustained success.

Building resilience assists employees in handling stress and encourages them to approach challenges with determination. Before we explore how to develop resilience, it's essential to understand why building it is important. Here are some benefits of being resilient in the workforce.

- **Aids job satisfaction:** Embracing resilience boosts job satisfaction. By using resilient approaches, you gain effective methods to handle stress and ease work-related anxiety. This not only improves your stress-coping skills but also fosters a sense of accomplishment and well-being in your professional journey. The positive effects extend throughout your work life, creating an overall feeling of fulfillment and contentment in your job. Resilience becomes a valuable tool, helping you overcome challenges and enhancing both your job satisfaction and personal well-being.

- **Improves employee self-esteem:** Strengthening your resilience can boost your self-esteem at work. Facing challenges with confidence and a positive mindset helps you overcome obstacles and builds a sense of accomplishment. This contributes to an improved self-image and a stronger belief in your abilities. Your resilient attitude creates a positive cycle, where each successfully managed challenge reinforces your self-esteem. It empowers you to confront workplace hurdles with positivity, resulting in increased confidence and a heightened sense of self-worth. This newfound assurance becomes a valuable asset, positively impacting not only your professional success but also your overall health.

- **Increases employee engagement:** Recognizing that work challenges are more manageable with the support of your colleagues is key. By appreciating the strength of collective support, you contribute to a collaborative and uplifting work environment. Your resilience becomes a shared asset, fostering camaraderie as colleagues unite to overcome challenges. In this supportive atmosphere, you not only improve your own ability to tackle work hurdles but also enhance the overall positivity and unity of the team.

- **Frames challenges as lessons:** In your work, a resilient mindset helps you see challenges as opportunities for skill-building and learning. Accepting that workplace challenges contribute to personal and professional growth allows you to turn difficulties into steps for improvement. This mindset empowers you to learn from experiences and enhance your skills continuously. Your resilience becomes a driving force, guiding you to face challenges with a growth-oriented mindset, contributing to a culture of continuous learning at your workplace.

- **Improves communication:** In your role, resilience empowers you to accept feedback openly, handle conflicts constructively, and contribute to a positive workplace culture. Approaching feedback with an open mindset demonstrates adaptability, fostering collaboration and understanding. This creates an atmosphere where diverse perspectives are embraced, and challenges are addressed with a collective commitment to growth and cooperation. By incorporating resilience into your interactions, you enhance professional relationships and contribute to the overall harmony and effectiveness of the team.

- **Supports innovation:** As someone with resilience, you likely find comfort in the concept of failure. This comfort empowers you to be open to taking well-informed risks in the workplace. You may explore new initiatives, share innovative ideas, and even take the lead on team projects. Embracing the idea that failure is a part of growth allows you to step outside your comfort zone and contribute to a culture of innovation within your workplace. Your openness to taking calculated risks becomes not only a testament to your resilience but also a driving force behind positive change and progress within the team and the organization as a whole.

- **Increases productivity:** Employees with resilience can support their colleagues, contributing to team success in the workplace. The overall productivity of a team or organization improves when mutual support exists among employees. For instance, team members facing challenges in a project can rely on each other for assistance. Collaborative efforts among coworkers lead to more efficient completion of team projects or tasks.

- **Creates leaders:** Leaders often possess resilience as a core characteristic, allowing them to overcome challenges effectively. When a workplace promotes resilience in its leaders, it sets positive examples for employees. These resilient leaders swiftly recover from mistakes and challenges, keeping employees motivated and preparing them for future leadership roles.

- **Encourages adaptability:** Resilience motivates individuals to embrace and adapt to changes. This skill is important as it empowers employees to swiftly adjust to workplace changes, minimizing disruptions and facilitating a smooth return to work. Consider a scenario where a company implements an innovative technology or software system that significantly changes the way tasks are managed. Resilient employees can easily adjust their work processes and learn to navigate the new system efficiently. Their ability to adapt and embrace technological changes ensures a seamless transition, allowing them to maintain the quality of their work despite the shift in tools and processes.

BUILDING PERSONAL RESILIENCE

If you want to become more adaptable and confident at work, consider implementing the following tips:

- **Develop positive habits:** Ensuring a healthy work-life balance and dedicating time for self-care can contribute to maintaining a positive mindset at work. Prioritize getting sufficient sleep and effectively managing stress to enhance your overall well-being. For instance, setting boundaries on work hours and incorporating activities you enjoy into your routine, such as regular exercise or hobbies, can significantly improve your work-life balance and positively impact your mindset. Taking these steps supports not only your professional performance but also your overall happiness and fulfillment.

- **Reflect on challenges:** When you handle a tough situation at work, take a moment to reflect and journal for future knowledge. Think about what aspects of the situation triggered your emotions and which decisions helped you overcome the challenge. For example, if you faced a tight project deadline, consider how time constraints impacted your stress levels. Identify strategies that worked, like prioritizing tasks or seeking support from colleagues.

- **Embrace a positive attitude:** Strive to arrive at work with a positive attitude, ready to collaborate with your teammates. The more enthusiasm and engagement you bring to your tasks, the more effectively you can navigate unforeseen circumstances. Imagine you have a team meeting to discuss a new project. Approach the meeting with an optimistic mindset, expressing eagerness to contribute ideas and work collaboratively. Your enthusiasm can inspire a more dynamic and productive atmosphere, making it easier for the team to handle unexpected challenges that may arise during the project.

- **Build trust with your manager and colleagues:** In your workplace, you may encounter collective challenges that you navigate alongside your team and manager. Establishing one-on-one meetings and building stronger relationships with your colleagues can enhance your comfort level when it comes to taking risks and devising solutions together. For example, consider scheduling regular one-on-one meetings with team members to discuss project challenges. By developing stronger connections, you create a supportive environment that encourages open communication and collaborative problem-solving. This increased comfort level can lead to more effective teamwork and innovative solutions to shared challenges.

- **Focus on what's in your control:** Certain factors at work, such as other people's moods, macroeconomic conditions, or client requests, may impact you and could be beyond your control. It's important to remember that you are only accountable for how you respond to these circumstances. If a colleague is in a bad mood, you can't control their emotions. Still, you can choose to respond with empathy and understanding rather than letting it negatively affect your own mood or productivity. Taking responsibility for your reactions allows you to maintain a positive and initiative-taking approach, even in situations beyond your control.

- **Take breaks:** In your journey to build resilience, it's vital to manage overwhelm and prevent burnout. Ensure you take regular breaks throughout your workday and make the most of any time off you receive to rest and disconnect from work. For instance, during your workday, schedule short breaks to recharge, whether it's a brief walk or a moment of relaxation. When you have time off, use it wisely to rejuvenate and step away from work-related responsibilities. Balancing your workload with restful breaks contributes to maintaining resilience and well- being in the long run.

BUILDING RESILIENCE AS A LEADER

For managers or executives seeking to enhance their team's resilience in the workplace, consider employing the following tips.

1. Set a positive example

In a workplace that promotes resilience, having leaders who exemplify this trait can be beneficial for you. Witnessing resilience in action on a daily basis can serve as a positive example, inspiring you to enhance your own resilience at work. When leading or collaborating with others, you can demonstrate strong leadership skills and resilience by setting workplace priorities, confronting challenges with confidence, and managing stress constructively.

2. Consider resilience training

Introducing resilience training in your workplace can provide you and your team with valuable tools to manage stress positively, address challenges professionally, and bounce back after facing difficulties. Seek out motivational experts who can inspire your team and teach them resilience-building techniques. Alternatively, encourage your colleagues and team members to create presentations sharing how they utilize this skill at work. Throughout the training, engage in discussions about the importance of resilience in the workplace and explore practical strategies for building and strengthening this valuable skill.

3. Learn more about employees' needs

As a manager, you can support your team members in building resilience by understanding their needs and identifying areas for improvement. Recognizing these challenges is crucial as resilience aims to strengthen individuals by enabling them to face and overcome obstacles. By understanding the specific obstacles, distractions, or challenges your employees encounter, you can develop strategies to assist them in overcoming these issues. To gather insights into your employees' needs, consider asking them to complete surveys detailing their challenges or provide opportunities for open discussions in one-on-one meetings. Armed with this information, you can then formulate plans to cultivate resilience and promote a positive work environment for everyone on the team.

4. Acknowledge failures

As a supervisor, when you acknowledge failures in the workplace, you play a key role in helping your team recognize and accept mistakes or issues objectively. This approach promotes resilience by providing support during challenging times and framing mistakes as neutral occurrences. Addressing failures involves encouraging employees to learn from their mistakes and use any disappointment as motivation. This motivation empowers them to move beyond their mistakes and make improvements for future success. By fostering an environment where employees accept and work through failures, you contribute to building self-resilience within the workplace.

5. Offer incentives to volunteer

As an employee, volunteering in the workplace provides you with a chance to challenge yourself and venture beyond your comfort zone. Embracing new or challenging projects and tasks during these opportunities can contribute to building your resilience. You might find yourself more motivated to seize these chances when your managers or team leaders provide incentives. For instance, consider the appeal of an extra day of paid time off for those who volunteer to lead and organize a project, requiring them to step up and take on additional responsibilities. This not only encourages personal growth but also fosters a resilient and proactive mindset within the workplace.

STRESS-RELIEF STRATEGIES FOR EMPLOYEES

As an employer, providing stress-relief opportunities for your employees is a valuable strategy to build resilience, offering them crucial time for recovery between projects. Here are some stress-relief outlets that you, as a team leader or manager, can incorporate into the workplace:

- **Offer wellness training:** Consider organizing wellness classes to guide your team members in stress relief techniques. You can encourage these habits by scheduling classes before or after work or even during lunch breaks. This proactive approach aims to promote your team members' well-being and resilience by equipping them with practical tools to manage and alleviate stress.

- **Coordinate support groups:** Encourage the formation of support groups in your workplace, allowing you and your colleagues to share challenges and provide mutual encouragement. When you support each other, it boosts your confidence in facing workplace challenges. This sense of camaraderie and shared support contributes to creating a positive and resilient work environment for all.

- **Enable workplace flexibility:** You can implement more flexible work arrangements, such as opportunities to work from home or take half-days. Providing you and your colleagues with increased flexibility or supporting your ability to take breaks can be instrumental in reducing stress and preventing burnout.

- **Play relaxing music:** In your workplace, playing relaxing music can contribute to creating a calmer environment for you and your colleagues. When you feel relaxed, it has the potential to reduce stress. Depending on the setting, managers may choose to play music in lunchrooms, break rooms, or lobbies to enhance the overall atmosphere.

- **Encourage affirmations:** In your workplace, affirmations can play a role in building your confidence and promoting positive thinking. Managers may display signs or posters throughout the office with helpful and positive affirmations or send affirmations to you and your team members via email.

Chapter 7
Creating Supportive Work Environments

To break free from Imposter Syndrome in the corporate world, you must begin with creating a supportive work environment. A positive and nurturing workplace contributes not only to a healthy mind but also to overall well-being, ultimately enhancing the quality of work produced. When employees feel mentally satisfied in their work environment, they are more likely to invest their best efforts into projects, fostering productivity and success. Prioritizing mental health creates a positive cycle, making individuals feel valued and motivated. This positive impact extends to both their professional performance and the overall work environment.

When employees see their needs are met, a reciprocal atmosphere emerges, and they are more likely to cater to the organization's needs. Working in a toxic environment is undesirable as it can adversely affect mental health. The strain from work-induced mental stress can also take a toll on physical well-being. When employees experience mental stress, it not only affects their work but can lead to health issues, resulting in potential delays due to illness. A healthy work environment enhances productivity and reduces the likelihood of disruptions caused by health-related absences.

As a leader, the implementation of healthy habits to foster a thriving environment may pose challenges. Establishing a flourishing workplace involves understanding and implementing practices that promote well-being among team members. It requires creating a culture where healthy habits are not only encouraged but also seamlessly integrated into daily routines. Leading by example, providing resources, and fostering open communication are key components in the journey toward establishing a work environment that nurtures the holistic health and success of every individual.

Work environments include the setting, social dynamics, and physical conditions of where you work. It affects key factors like morale, relationships, performance, job satisfaction, and health. Knowing what defines a work environment and what makes it healthy can guide your choice of employers. A positive work environment brightens the mood, improves concentration, and provides a good working approach for both employees and employers. The workplace's physical layout, the tools and equipment used, ambient noise and lighting, the allowance for listening to music, temperature, and ventilation, as well as safety and security measures - all these factors play a crucial role.

Beyond these physical aspects, the workplace environment includes social and cultural elements. This involves organizational culture, communication style, relationships among colleagues and supervisors, and the level of support and recognition offered to employees.

Supportive environments boost productivity, creativity, and employee satisfaction. It is characterized by clear communication, effective teamwork, diversity, respect, and a commitment to employee concerns. Conversely, a negative workplace environment can lead to occupational stress, burnout, and low morale, impacting both individual and organizational performance.

Here are some ways leaders can address and support employee mental health. These approaches contribute to creating a supportive work environment, making it easier for everyone to coexist.

1. Make sure you're as well-staffed as possible.

Amid staffing shortages and competitive employment opportunities, numerous businesses are functioning with a minimal workforce. Consequently, those present are compelled to handle additional tasks and assume greater responsibilities. The burdensome workloads and the expectation to work faster and longer hours frequently result in physical and mental health challenges, issues that could be settled down with sufficient staffing.

If your team is understaffed, it is necessary to reconsider and enhance compensation and other factors to attract talent. Without addressing these concerns, valued employees may eventually experience burnout or develop resentment, potentially leading to leaving. By prioritizing employee well-being, acknowledging their contributions, and fostering a collaborative atmosphere, organizations can cultivate a workforce that is not only abundant in numbers but also empowered, confident, and less susceptible to the detrimental effects of Imposter Syndrome.

2. Create a schedule for stability and work consistency.

In crafting a schedule for stability and work consistency, it is essential to weave the fabric of a supportive work environment, recognizing its pivotal role in fortifying against Imposter Syndrome. One critical aspect is fostering open lines of communication within the workplace. Establishing clear channels for feedback and dialogue helps in articulating expectations, providing constructive criticism, and creating an atmosphere where employees feel heard and acknowledged. Regular team meetings, one-on-one sessions, and performance reviews contribute to this dialogue, allowing individuals to discuss their concerns, seek guidance, and receive reassurance about their contributions. This transparent communication not only enhances clarity regarding job roles and responsibilities but also plays a crucial role in dismantling the self-doubt that often characterizes Imposter Syndrome.

Moreover, a supportive work environment goes hand in hand with the cultivation of a culture that prioritizes employee well-being. Organizations can implement flexible work schedules, remote work options, and wellness programs to accommodate the diverse needs of their workforce. By acknowledging the importance of work-life balance, companies not only contribute to the stability of their employees but also create an environment that is less conducive to the development of Imposter Syndrome. Encouraging a healthy work-life integration not only enhances job satisfaction but also bolsters confidence by validating the significance of personal well-being alongside professional success. As employees witness a genuine commitment to their holistic development, they are more likely to feel secure, supported, and empowered in their roles, fostering an environment conducive to sustained stability and work consistency.

3. Empower employees with freedom.

Empowering employees with the freedom to excel within a supportive work environment is a strategic approach to not only boost productivity but also to counteract the insidious effects of Imposter Syndrome. An essential aspect of this empowerment is entrusting employees with autonomy in decision-making. Allowing individuals to make choices and contribute their unique perspectives fosters a sense of ownership and confidence in their abilities. This autonomy extends beyond daily tasks to encompass project management, goal setting, and problem-solving. By relinquishing a certain level of control and encouraging self-direction, organizations cultivate a culture that values individual strengths, fostering an environment where employees are less likely to succumb to feelings of inadequacy associated with Imposter Syndrome.

In addition to autonomy, providing opportunities for skill development and continuous learning is a potent tool for empowerment. A supportive work environment invests in the growth of its employees through training programs, mentorship initiatives, and professional development opportunities. This not only enhances their expertise but also sends a clear message that the organization believes in their potential. By acquiring new skills and expanding their knowledge base, employees feel better equipped to navigate challenges, reducing the likelihood of experiencing Imposter Syndrome. This empowerment through education not only enhances job satisfaction but also builds a resilient and confident workforce, capable of tackling complex tasks and contributing meaningfully to the organization's success. In essence, by fostering a culture that empowers employees, organizations create a potent antidote to the pervasive effects of Imposter Syndrome, ensuring a more confident and capable workforce.

4. Allow for more flexibility in when and where employees work.

Introducing greater flexibility in terms of when and where employees work is a strategic initiative that not only embraces the evolving nature of work but also contributes significantly to the creation of a supportive environment that can alleviate the effects of Imposter Syndrome. By allowing employees to set their work hours or adopt remote work options, organizations acknowledge the diverse needs and lifestyles of their workforce. This flexibility demonstrates a level of trust in employees' ability to manage their responsibilities autonomously, fostering a sense of empowerment that acts as a powerful counterforce to Imposter Syndrome. Moreover, flexible work arrangements enable individuals to create a personalized work environment that enhances their productivity and overall job satisfaction, reducing the likelihood of feeling undeserving of their roles.

In addition to flexibility in work hours and location, a supportive work environment should actively promote work-life balance. Encouraging employees to take breaks, use vacation time, and prioritize their well-being sends a clear message that their mental and emotional health is valued. This approach is particularly crucial in mitigating Imposter Syndrome, as individuals often grapple with feelings of inadequacy when the boundary between work and personal life blurs. A workplace that values and supports a healthy balance between professional and personal pursuits contributes to a more resilient and content workforce. By cultivating an environment that understands and accommodates the individual needs of employees, organizations not only enhance their overall work culture but also create a buffer against the psychological challenges associated with Imposter Syndrome.

5. Extend more grace when personal needs arise.

Extending more grace when personal needs arise is a cornerstone of creating a supportive work environment that plays a pivotal role in mitigating the impacts of Imposter Syndrome. Recognizing and accommodating the personal challenges and needs of employees demonstrates a profound understanding of their humanity beyond their professional roles. This involves fostering a culture that values empathy and compassion, allowing individuals to navigate personal circumstances without fear of judgment or repercussions. By acknowledging that everyone encounters unforeseen personal challenges, from family emergencies to health issues, organizations contribute to an atmosphere where employees feel supported rather than burdened by their personal lives. This empathetic approach not only builds trust but also helps dismantle the negative thought patterns associated with Imposter Syndrome, as individuals feel reassured that their worth is not solely tied to their professional output.

Moreover, encouraging open communication about personal needs creates a culture of transparency and trust. When employees feel comfortable discussing their personal challenges, it enables the organization to provide the necessary support and accommodations. This might involve flexible work hours, temporary workload adjustments, or access to mental health resources. In turn, this approach not only helps individuals navigate personal crises but also reinforces a sense of belonging within the workplace. By fostering an environment where employees are seen as whole individuals with multifaceted lives, organizations contribute to a resilient workforce less susceptible to the doubts and insecurities associated with Imposter Syndrome. In essence, extending grace in the face of personal needs is a proactive strategy for building a workplace that prioritizes the well-being of its employees, ultimately creating a robust defense against the psychological challenges that can hinder professional confidence.

6. Cultivate inclusivity and a sense of belonging.

Cultivating inclusivity and fostering a sense of belonging is a foundational strategy for creating a supportive work environment that significantly contributes to the alleviation of Imposter Syndrome among employees. Inclusive practices involve going beyond diversity quotas and actively seeking to understand, respect, and celebrate the unique backgrounds and perspectives of each individual within the organization. Establishing inclusive policies and initiatives not only breaks down barriers to entry but also ensures that all employees feel valued and heard. A workplace that actively cultivates inclusivity sends a powerful message that diverse voices are not only welcome but essential for the organization's success. By creating an environment where individuals can bring their authentic selves to work, organizations provide a powerful antidote to the feelings of inadequacy and self-doubt associated with Imposter Syndrome.

Furthermore, promoting a sense of belonging is integral to combating Imposter Syndrome. Employees who feel connected to their colleagues and the organization are more likely to experience a positive self-perception and confidence in their abilities. This can be achieved through team-building activities, mentorship programs, and initiatives that encourage collaboration. When individuals feel a sense of community and support, they are less likely to attribute their success to luck or external factors, addressing the core issues that underlie Imposter Syndrome. Organizations can also establish affinity groups or employee resource networks that provide a platform for shared experiences and mutual support. In creating an environment where everyone feels valued and connected, organizations not only enhance employee well-being but also foster a workforce that is more resilient and less susceptible to the psychological challenges associated with Imposter Syndrome.

7. Provide growth and development opportunities.

Providing ample growth and development opportunities within a supportive work environment is a cornerstone strategy for mitigating the effects of Imposter Syndrome and fostering a culture of professional empowerment. This involves investing in ongoing training programs, skill-building workshops, and mentorship initiatives that cater to the diverse needs and aspirations of employees. By offering avenues for continuous learning and career advancement, organizations not only enhance the capabilities of their workforce but also send a powerful message that individual growth is prioritized. This proactive approach directly combats the feelings of self-doubt associated with Imposter Syndrome, as employees witness tangible support for their professional development, affirming their competence and potential.

In addition to formalized training, organizations can create a supportive atmosphere that encourages employees to explore new roles, take on challenging projects, and participate in cross-functional collaborations. This approach allows individuals to stretch their capabilities and step outside their comfort zones, fostering a sense of accomplishment and mastery that counteracts the negative thought patterns linked to Imposter Syndrome. Moreover, mentorship programs provide guidance and support, offering individuals a trusted source of advice and encouragement. As employees receive acknowledgment for their achievements and witness their progression within the organization, they are more likely to build a resilient self-image, less susceptible to the feelings of fraudulence that often characterize Imposter Syndrome. Overall, by actively promoting growth and development opportunities, organizations not only enhance the skill sets of their workforce but also contribute to a workplace culture that bolsters confidence and diminishes the impact of Imposter Syndrome.

8. Advocate for paid time off and benefits utilization.

Advocating for paid time off (PTO) and encouraging the utilization of benefits is a crucial component in creating a supportive work environment that can significantly contribute to the improvement of Imposter Syndrome among employees. Acknowledging the importance of work-life balance, organizations that prioritize and advocate for PTO recognize the need for employees to recharge and attend to personal matters without the burden of guilt or apprehension. This advocacy sends a powerful message that the organization values the holistic well-being of its workforce, promoting a culture that understands the significance of rest and rejuvenation. By actively encouraging employees to take advantage of their allocated time off, organizations contribute to the reduction of burnout and stress, both of which are contributing factors to Imposter Syndrome. A well-rested and balanced workforce is better equipped to navigate challenges with confidence and resilience.

Furthermore, promoting the utilization of benefits beyond just PTO, such as health and wellness programs, mental health resources, and family support initiatives, contributes to a comprehensive strategy in fostering a supportive work environment. These benefits not only address the physical and mental well-being of employees but also underscore the organization's commitment to their overall quality of life. When employees feel supported in various aspects of their lives, they are less likely to succumb to the negative thought patterns associated with Imposter Syndrome. This approach goes beyond mere lip service to employee well-being; it actively demonstrates a commitment to creating a workplace where individuals feel valued, cared for, and capable. In essence, advocating for PTO and comprehensive benefits utilization is a proactive step towards creating an environment that empowers employees and mitigates the psychological challenges associated with Imposter Syndrome.

9. Encourage movement, fitness, and healthy habits.

Encouraging movement, fitness, and healthy habits within the workplace is a transformative strategy for creating a supportive environment that holds the potential to significantly improve Imposter Syndrome among employees. By fostering a culture that prioritizes physical well-being, organizations signal a commitment to the holistic health of their workforce. This can be achieved by providing on-site fitness facilities, organizing wellness programs, or even instituting policies that promote regular breaks for physical activity. Engaging in regular exercise has been proven to reduce stress, boost mood, and enhance cognitive function—all factors that contribute to a more resilient mindset. When employees are encouraged to incorporate movement into their daily routines, they are better equipped to manage the mental and emotional challenges that can manifest as Imposter Syndrome.

Moreover, initiatives that encourage healthy habits extend beyond the physical realm, encompassing mental and emotional well-being as well. Offering mindfulness and stress-management programs, promoting flexible work hours to accommodate personal wellness practices, and providing resources for mental health support contribute to a more comprehensive approach. As individuals adopt healthier habits, they are more likely to develop a positive self-image and greater resilience in the face of challenges. This, in turn, directly counters the feelings of self-doubt and inadequacy associated with Imposter Syndrome. In creating an environment that not only values but actively promotes physical and mental well-being, organizations foster a workplace culture that not only enhances the overall health of their employees but also acts as a buffer against the psychological toll of Imposter Syndrome.

10. Spread positivity.

Spreading positivity is a foundational pillar in the creation of a supportive work environment, and it plays a significant role in improving Imposter Syndrome among employees. Encouraging a positive atmosphere involves not only recognizing and celebrating achievements but also fostering a culture of constructive feedback. By focusing on strengths and accomplishments, organizations can create a workplace where individuals feel acknowledged and valued, diminishing the tendency to attribute success to luck or external factors—a common manifestation of Imposter Syndrome. Regularly highlighting accomplishments, whether big or small, contributes to a positive narrative that shapes employees' self-perception and bolsters their confidence.

In addition to recognizing achievements, promoting a culture of gratitude and appreciation further enhances positivity in the workplace. Simple gestures such as expressing gratitude for team efforts, acknowledging hard work, and celebrating milestones create an environment where employees feel seen and appreciated. This positive reinforcement contributes to a sense of belonging and reduces the likelihood of individuals feeling like impostors in their roles. Positivity is contagious, and when it becomes a pervasive aspect of the work culture, it acts as a powerful buffer against the negative thought patterns associated with Imposter Syndrome. Employees in such an environment are more likely to support each other, collaborate effectively, and navigate challenges with a mindset focused on growth and achievement.

Furthermore, leadership plays a crucial role in setting the tone for positivity within the workplace. Leaders who exemplify optimism, resilience, and a constructive approach to problem-solving create a ripple effect that permeates the entire organization. Transparent and open communication from leadership fosters a climate of trust and psychological safety, essential elements in combatting Imposter Syndrome. When employees feel supported by their leaders, they are more likely to view challenges as opportunities for growth rather than as threats to their competence. Leadership that actively promotes a positive work culture sends a clear message that mistakes are viewed as learning experiences, not as indicators of incompetence, thus addressing one of the root causes of Imposter Syndrome.

Lastly, incorporating activities that promote well-being and camaraderie can contribute significantly to a positive work environment. Organizing team-building events, social gatherings, and wellness initiatives not only enhance the overall workplace experience but also create opportunities for employees to connect on a personal level. A sense of camaraderie and shared purpose helps individuals feel supported and less isolated in their experiences. Social connections and positive relationships act as a powerful antidote to Imposter Syndrome by reinforcing a sense of belonging and mutual support.

In conclusion, spreading positivity within the workplace is a multifaceted approach that involves recognizing achievements, expressing gratitude, fostering leadership that exemplifies optimism, and promoting social connections. By actively cultivating a positive work culture, organizations can create an environment where employees feel empowered, valued, and less susceptible to the detrimental effects of Imposter Syndrome.

ADVOCATING FOR CHANGE IN YOUR WORKPLACE

Advocating for change in the workplace to create a supportive environment is not just a noble pursuit; it is a strategic imperative, particularly in the context of combating Imposter Syndrome. This initiative requires a holistic and intentional approach that addresses various facets of the organizational culture, policies, and leadership dynamics. By actively championing change, individuals and organizations can contribute significantly to alleviating the psychological burden of Imposter Syndrome among employees.

A crucial aspect of advocating for change is challenging traditional notions of success and competence. This involves moving away from a culture that places undue emphasis on perfectionism and recognizing that setbacks and mistakes are integral to the learning process. By fostering an environment that views failures as opportunities for growth, individuals are less likely to succumb to the pervasive self-doubt associated with Imposter Syndrome. Advocating for this cultural shift encourages a mindset focused on resilience and continuous improvement, creating a workplace where employees feel empowered to take risks and learn from their experiences.

In the pursuit of change, organizations must also prioritize diversity, equity, and inclusion. Promoting a workplace that is genuinely diverse and inclusive is instrumental in dismantling the stereotypes and biases that contribute to Imposter

Syndrome. Advocating for diverse hiring practices, providing equal opportunities for advancement, and fostering an inclusive culture where every voice is heard are critical steps in creating an environment where individuals from various backgrounds feel valued and supported. As workplace diversity increases, individuals are less likely to attribute their success to external factors, reducing the prevalence of Imposter Syndrome.

Leadership plays a pivotal role in driving change within the workplace. Advocating for a leadership style that emphasizes empathy, transparency, and mentorship creates a supportive environment that directly addresses the root causes of Imposter Syndrome. Leaders who openly share their experiences of overcoming challenges and acknowledge their vulnerabilities set a precedent that vulnerability is not synonymous with weakness. Such leaders become role models for authenticity, demonstrating that it is acceptable to be imperfect and that success does not require a façade of infallibility. Advocating for leadership that prioritizes mentorship and coaching further supports individuals in their professional development, offering guidance and reassurance that is instrumental in mitigating the effects of Imposter Syndrome.

Moreover, advocating for change involves reshaping performance evaluations and feedback mechanisms. Implementing a system that emphasizes constructive feedback over criticism fosters an environment where employees feel supported in their growth. Regular, transparent communication about expectations, progress, and areas for improvement contributes to a workplace culture that values continuous learning rather than perfection. This shift in evaluation methods directly addresses the fear of falling short and not meeting expectations—a common trigger for Imposter Syndrome.

In the realm of mental health, advocating for change includes destigmatizing discussions around well-being. Encouraging open conversations about mental health, providing access to resources such as counseling services, and integrating mental health initiatives into the workplace create an environment where individuals feel comfortable addressing their psychological well-being. As mental health becomes a normalized topic, the shame and secrecy associated with Imposter Syndrome are diminished, and individuals are more likely to seek support and share their experiences.

In conclusion, advocating for change in the workplace to create a supportive environment is a multifaceted and transformative endeavor. By challenging traditional notions of success, prioritizing diversity and inclusion, promoting authentic leadership, reshaping performance evaluations, and destigmatizing mental health discussions, organizations can actively contribute to the reduction of Imposter Syndrome. This advocacy not only enhances the well-being of individual employees but also fosters a workplace culture that values authenticity, resilience, and continuous growth. Ultimately, the positive impact of these changes extends beyond the professional realm, creating an environment where individuals can thrive personally and professionally, free from the shackles of Imposter Syndrome.

Chapter 8
Diversity and Inclusion in the Workplace

In a workplace that prioritizes diversity and inclusivity, the experience of equal involvement and support is crucial to combating Imposter Syndrome. Regardless of your background or role within the organization, this commitment ensures that you feel included and supported in all aspects of your professional journey. The celebration of unique contributions fosters an environment where every voice is heard and respected, contributing to the collective success of the entire team.

However, Imposter Syndrome can thrive in environments where diversity and inclusion are not fully integrated across all levels and facets of the workplace. It's not just about having a diverse workforce but ensuring that diversity is present in leadership roles as well. Without this integration, individuals may feel a sense of inadequacy or doubt about their abilities, contributing to Imposter Syndrome.

Inclusive efforts should specifically concentrate on making every employee, regardless of their background, feel appreciated and trusted. This involves recognizing and accommodating the unique needs and practices of individuals, ensuring that their voices are considered equal to others. When employees feel the need to conceal or alter essential aspects of themselves, it significantly impacts job satisfaction and can contribute to higher rates of Imposter Syndrome.

Acknowledging and honoring diverse religious and cultural practices is a key component of fostering inclusion. This involves not only recognizing but actively accommodating these practices through policies that support flexible scheduling, designated spaces for prayer or meditation, and time off for significant cultural or religious holidays. By celebrating a variety of festivals and traditions, organizations can demonstrate their commitment to diversity and create an environment where everyone feels supported in practicing their beliefs.

Employee retention is directly linked to how individuals perceive their organization's commitment to diversity and inclusion. Creating a workplace where every voice is welcomed, listened to, and respected helps establish a genuine connection to the company. When employees feel included and accepted for who they are, regardless of various factors like age, gender, or cultural background, it fosters a sense of belonging and helps combat Imposter Syndrome.

Investing in a workforce communications platform is a practical step toward fostering inclusion. This platform ensures that communication channels are integrated, reaching each worker through their preferred medium. This not only aids in connection but also gathers insights through unified analytics, supporting a more personalized and inclusive employee experience.

Transparent discussions about gender and potential pay disparities contribute to building trust and inclusivity. By openly addressing gender pay imbalances and sharing strategies to bridge the gap, companies demonstrate a commitment to fairness and equality. Transparent communication, as exemplified by companies like Microsoft under CEO Satya Nadella, sets an example for fostering a culture of openness and accountability. This proactive approach helps in addressing concerns, building trust, and actively combating Imposter Syndrome in the workplace.

Welcome a multilingual workforce.

Imagine navigating a workplace where the predominant language is not your native tongue, a scenario ripe for triggering Imposter Syndrome. In this inclusive environment, the celebration of diverse languages and cultures creates a dynamic atmosphere where the unique linguistic background of each individual is not just acknowledged but genuinely valued.

To counteract Imposter Syndrome, it's crucial to be mindful of language barriers and preferences, especially in global companies with diverse teams spread across different countries. Even when a common language is used, decisions about language choices for events become pivotal. Reflect on the inclusivity of language during virtual events—what language will the CEO choose for their speech? Thoughtful decisions in these situations promote a sense of inclusion, ensuring that everyone, regardless of their linguistic background, feels valued and understood.

In larger global companies, providing translation services is a key practice to foster understanding and inclusion. However, in smaller companies, prioritizing everyday employee comfort in communication is equally vital. This involves creating an environment where employees feel at ease using their preferred language, particularly in common areas or during company-sponsored events, thus mitigating the potential triggers of Imposter Syndrome.

As a strategic approach to combat Imposter Syndrome in the long term, cultivating a multilingual workforce can be a transformative investment. This may involve offering educational opportunities for employees to learn additional languages. While this might seem initially costly, consider it an investment that not only enriches the linguistic diversity of the workplace but also yields significant returns over time in terms of employee satisfaction and overall well-being.

Foster diverse thinking

When you proactively incorporate diversity into your hiring practices, you position your company to welcome a myriad of culturally diverse perspectives. Yet, for these varied viewpoints to truly flourish, it's imperative to prioritize inclusivity within your workplace culture, especially in the context of combating Imposter Syndrome.

Recognizing the significance of diversity becomes essential as individuals from diverse backgrounds and generations bring markedly different perspectives to various aspects of work. This divergence extends beyond superficial aspects like clothing choices and email composition, seeping into the feedback shared in employee reviews and the ideas presented in meetings. It's not just crucial for individual employees, small teams, or departments to comprehend these thinking patterns; understanding how others across the entire company think is equally important. This broader understanding cultivates a collaborative and inclusive environment where diverse viewpoints contribute to the overall creativity and success of the organization, helping counteract the isolating effects of Imposter Syndrome.

Embracing diverse thinking proves valuable in generating innovative ideas and receiving constructive feedback, all while creating an environment where everyone feels relevant and part of a shared mission.

Pixar Animation Studios stands as an exemplary model of a company successfully embracing diverse thinking. Ed Catmull, the co-founder and president of Pixar, underscores the importance of fostering a culture that encourages diverse perspectives in his book "Creativity, Inc."

At Pixar, the creative process involves collaborative input from individuals with diverse backgrounds, experiences, and expertise. The company acknowledges that diverse thinking is indispensable for creating innovative and engaging storytelling. For example, during the development of the movie "Coco," centered around Mexican culture and traditions, Pixar established a "Cultural Trust" comprising external experts and cultural consultants to ensure an authentic representation.

By actively seeking diverse perspectives, Pixar consistently produces critically acclaimed and commercially successful films. The emphasis on embracing diverse thinking not only results in creative and original ideas but also establishes an inclusive environment where everyone's contributions are valued. This approach significantly contributes to Pixar's success in storytelling and animation, illustrating the effectiveness of embracing diverse perspectives in the creative process and its relevance in alleviating Imposter Syndrome.

Embracing Multigenerational Diversity

In the contemporary workforce, millennials dominate, underscoring the imperative for a workplace that not only acknowledges but actively accommodates multiple generations. Creating a diverse and inclusive workforce requires a nuanced understanding of millennials, a group born from 1981 onwards, acknowledging their diversity beyond the common association with tech-savviness. It's crucial to recognize that older millennials may not possess the same proficiency with technology tools as their younger counterparts.

These generational differences manifest in various aspects, especially in communication practices within the workplace. While some employees, particularly millennials, may prefer utilizing social channels or group chats, individuals from older generations might not readily embrace these communication platforms. To bridge this communication gap, investing in a workforce communications platform becomes paramount. This tool streamlines the creation and efficient delivery of messages through various channels, catering to the diverse preferences present across generations within the workforce.

In the context of combating Imposter Syndrome, acknowledging and accommodating these generational differences contributes to fostering an inclusive environment. It ensures that individuals, regardless of their age or technological proficiency, feel valued and included in the communication processes of the organization, thereby mitigating potential triggers of Imposter Syndrome.

Eliminate bias in the appraisal process and promotion opportunities.

In numerous instances, hiring processes have been identified as unfair and lengthy, marred by unconscious biases such as sexism, racism, and ageism. The unchecked prevalence of these biases poses a significant threat to your company. When certain roles are conventionally associated with specific genders or age groups, it leads to the application of different standards in hiring, promoting, and evaluating job performance. For instance, the absence of male kindergarten teachers or female engineers can reinforce stereotypes, affecting decision-making in recruitment and career advancement. Addressing these biases becomes paramount for creating a workplace environment that actively combats Imposter Syndrome, ensuring talent is recognized and rewarded without regard to gender, race, or age.

Managers play a pivotal role in learning and implementing practices that actively counteract biases in procedures. By adopting such measures, you contribute to the establishment of a more equitable and inclusive workplace, thus mitigating the potential triggers of Imposter Syndrome.

Some effective strategies to combat bias include:

• Rewriting Job Descriptions: Ensure job descriptions are gender-neutral, using language that strikes a balance of gendered descriptors and verbs, fostering a more inclusive perception of roles.

• Implementing Blind Resume Review: Create a blind system for reviewing resumes, eliminating visibility of demographic characteristics during the initial assessment to ensure fair and unbiased evaluations.

• Setting Diversity Goals: Establish organizational diversity goals to track and measure progress, promoting transparency and accountability in fostering a diverse and inclusive workplace.

By incorporating these strategies, managers actively contribute to breaking down unconscious biases, creating a work environment where talent and capabilities are acknowledged and rewarded based on merit rather than preconceived notions related to gender, race, or age. In turn, this helps in fostering an environment that actively combats Imposter Syndrome by providing an equal and fair platform for all employees to thrive

THE LINK BETWEEN IMPOSTER SYNDROME AND INCLUSION

The connection between imposter syndrome and inclusion is significant. Imposter syndrome can fuel feelings of exclusion and marginalization among those who struggle with it.

Suppose an individual perceives themselves as not fitting into a specific professional environment. In that case, they might hesitate to voice their opinions in meetings, leading to a heightened sense of isolation and disconnection from their peers.

On the other hand, an inclusive environment not only diminishes feelings of imposter syndrome but also cultivates a strong sense of belonging among individuals. When people experience acceptance and value for who they are, regardless of their background or identity, it naturally enhances their confidence in their abilities. Creating a culture of inclusion empowers individuals to be more self-assured and contributes to a positive and supportive workplace atmosphere.

One of the several causes of imposter syndrome that you may encounter is racial stereotyping. Historically, Black individuals, particularly males, have faced negative stereotypes regarding their intellectual abilities. Within institutions of higher learning, these biases can contribute to feelings of inadequacy, fostering a constant need to prove oneself in academic environments. Individuals must be aware of and challenge these stereotypes, fostering an environment where everyone is judged based on their merits rather than harmful preconceptions.

Another factor contributing to imposter syndrome that you might relate to is the absence of representation. When there's a shortage of role models and mentors who share the same racial background, it can generate feelings of isolation and self-doubt among Black students. The lack of representation makes visualizing success in certain fields challenging, heightening the likelihood of experiencing imposter syndrome within academic programs.

Moreover, discrimination and microaggressions are additional factors that may contribute to imposter syndrome. Encountering discrimination and subtle yet harmful microaggressions within academic programs can result in an overwhelming sense of exclusion and marginalization. The persistent exposure to such negative academic environments adds to the likelihood of experiencing Imposter Syndrome among Black students. This constant negativity can lead them to question their abilities, qualifications, and, ultimately, their presence in the programs.

Chapter 9
Case Studies and Interviews

Leaders frequently struggle with imposter syndrome. Even in the face of observable success and professional recognition, these emotions of hopelessness and self-doubt frequently endure. These feelings can be made worse by the pressure to perform well and uphold high standards, which can affect leaders in a variety of industries. Let's study some real-world leaders and imposter syndrome.

Case Study 1: Sheryl Sandberg

Take into consideration Sheryl Sandberg's experiences. She is the Chief Operating Officer of Facebook and the author of "Lean In." Even though Sandberg played an important part in creating one of the biggest internet firms in the world, she freely said that she struggled with self-doubt and the worry that she wasn't qualified for her role. Her openness about her battles with Imposter Syndrome has struck a chord with a great number of professionals throughout the world, demonstrating that even highly successful leaders struggle with feelings of self-worth.

Sandberg's career path was marked with achievements, but enduring emotions of imposter syndrome and self-doubt hampered her progress. She was an exceptionally bright child who went to Harvard University for her undergraduate education before going on to Harvard Business School to get her MBA. Her determination and academic prowess were apparent at a young age, letting her get into important positions in the public and commercial sectors.

An important turning point in Sandberg's career was when she joined Google in its early days. Her substantial contributions to Google's expansion cemented her standing as a skillful and astute leader. Even so, she battled self-doubt about her ability despite her achievements. She was clearly successful, yet this self-doubt, rooted in the imposter syndrome phenomena, persisted.

Sandberg shot into being internationally famous when she joined Facebook in 2008 and took on the COO position. She led the company through important stages of growth in both income and expansion during her time at the social networking site, which is just one of many impressive things she did there. Even so, she secretly struggled with feelings of being ineligible, believing that her position did not warrant her level of competence.

Her self-reflective story in "Lean In" openly discusses the internal struggles she had. Many aspirational leaders connected with Sandberg's openness regarding her battles with imposter syndrome. Despite her evident success in her achievements, this syndrome made her feel as if she was not enough.

However, she combated self-doubt. Her bravery in disclosing these inner battles illuminated how common imposter syndrome is, especially among successful executives.

Case Study 2: Howard Schultz

Now, let's take a look at the story of Howard Schultz's rise from Starbucks employee to CEO and his continuous struggle with imposter syndrome shows how he was affected.

The narrative of Schultz started in the early 1980s when he was hired as Director of Retail Operations and Marketing by Starbucks, a small local retailer of coffee beans at the time. Because of his forward-thinking viewpoint, he saw Starbucks as more than just a location to buy coffee; it could develop into a hub for the community and provide experiences beyond just coffee. His support of this idea ultimately resulted in the development of Starbucks cafés as we know them today.

Schultz struggled on the inside, even though he was dedicated to turning Starbucks into a worldwide brand. He achieved so many great things that people never doubted his skills. He was never hesitant to discuss his struggle with imposter syndrome and the feelings of unworthiness he always had while giving interviews and even in his autobiography, "Pour Your Heart Into It."

In his self-reflections, Schultz admitted that he had doubts when he thought that he actually deserved all these honors and all the success. He usually doubted himself, even when his leadership and decisions had great importance.

In his interviews, he talked about how afraid he was about not meeting the standards and how proud he was of what Starbucks had done. Schultz's body language and words showed that he was having a rough time within himself. This showed the duality of a great leader who has problems with self-doubt.

Though in the midst of these difficulties, Schultz's persistency helped Starbucks reach a high point. His steadfast faith in the company's potential and his dedication to creating a distinctive coffeehouse experience were crucial to its success on a worldwide scale.

Schultz did a lot of hard things on his trip, which shows how complicated his imposter syndrome was. Being worried all the time shows how imposter syndrome can affect even the most successful CEOs, despite the fact he made a small business into an international business. By talking about these problems, he gives the achievement story a human touch and shows how great people deal with problems on the inside.

Case Study 3: Indra Nooyi

Let's take a look at Indra Nooyi. She went from being a poor Indian girl to being the CEO of PepsiCo. This shows how strong, smart, and capable she is to lead a journey. She did have some problems along the way, though. The worst was that she had was also imposter syndrome.

Nooyi's career path was marked by academic success. She joined the Indian Institute of Management Calcutta with an MBA and later graduated from Yale School of Management with a Master's. She started out as a business leader by holding a number of senior positions at companies like Motorola and Asea Brown Boveri. It was there that she learned how to be smart about strategy.

After joining PepsiCo in 1994, Nooyi quickly moved up the company, showing how great a leader she is. She finally became CEO of PepsiCo in 2006 after leading important projects that helped the company grow and become more diverse.

Nooyi has discussed her battles with imposter syndrome in interviews and public engagements despite her incredible accomplishments. She talked of having self-doubt, feeling like an outsider in boardrooms, and worrying that she wouldn't live up to expectations.

Her observations on imposter syndrome were in line with the feelings of many successful people. Professionals from a variety of professions were moved by Nooyi's honesty about her inner struggles, which illuminated the emotional agony that can accompany accomplishment at the top echelons of corporate leadership.

Several techniques helped Nooyi get over her imposter feeling.

She underlined the value of tenacity and persistently looking for chances to learn and develop. Nooyi also placed a high value on mentoring, encircling herself with a network of friends and family, and asking peers and reliable experts for advice.

Nooyi also talked about how important it is to accept one's point of view and go against common ideas about leadership. She highlighted being honest and true to oneself, knowing that a leader could be both weak and strong at the same time.

Many people who want to be leaders looked up to Nooyi because she was honest about how she dealt with imposter syndrome while running a big global company like Pepsi. Her strength and strong approach to getting over her self-doubt teach us a lot about how to get over imposter syndrome in stressful work settings.

Case Study 4: Elon Musk

In addition to always coming up with new ideas, Elon Musk is known for being the CEO of game-changing companies like SpaceX, Tesla, and others. He is also known for being open about the fact that he struggles with imposter syndrome, even though he is a great leader.

Many people know Musk from his work with companies like Zip2 and PayPal, but what really made him famous was his wish to change the auto and space industries. His big ideas were shown by SpaceX's work in space research and Tesla's electric cars. Musk has been open about his struggles with imposter syndrome behind the scenes, though.

Musk has said in a number of public appearances and talks that he sometimes doubts his own abilities. Even though he did amazing things, the weight of responsibility and the close attention of the public often made him feel like he wasn't good enough. Musk's honesty about these problems makes him seem more likable, which makes him popular with people who want to be business owners and leaders.

A lot of his ideas about imposter syndrome are based on the huge stress that comes with making groundbreaking new technologies. Musk has said that he sometimes has doubts about his abilities and wonders if he can reach the crazy goals he sets for his businesses.

Musk fights the imposter syndrome in a number of different ways. His unshakable determination to push the limits and his strong work spirit help him deal with problems and keep him going. As a result of focusing on the technical aspects of his projects, Musk stayed responsible and skilled.

Musk also finds comfort in the understanding and skill of his staff. With the help of amazing people and faith in their abilities, he lowers his doubts. In addition, Musk fixes problems by facing problems head-on, which calms him down and restores his faith in his leadership skills.

Musk is willing to take risks and failure as a way to get over his imposter syndrome, which is interesting to note. He knows that mistakes are unavoidable and necessary for growth, but he also thinks that failures are important parts of the invention process.

Case Study 5: Maya Angelou

Furthermore, the famous author, poet, and civil rights fighter Maya Angelou changed literature and society in a way that will last for a long time. She told everyone that she had imposter syndrome, even though she was very talented and had won many awards. This brought attention to how common the condition is and how it affects people from every aspect of life.

Angelou's creative works, such as her groundbreaking autobiography "I Know Why the Caged Bird Sings," poem collections, and essays, were praised by critics and recognized around the world. But she also said in interviews and writings that she was insecure about herself and was afraid of being caught as fake.

Her ideas about imposter syndrome showed that even the most successful person could have doubts about their own skills. Angelou's truthfulness about these feelings touched a lot of people from all walks of life, showing how common and unspecific imposter syndrome is.

Angelou openly discussed her personal struggles in interviews and her autobiographical writings despite her outward achievements. She said she had times when she didn't believe in herself and wondered if she really achieved all the recognition and honors she had received. Her public image became more human when she talked about these problems. This made her a relatable figure for many people who want to be successful in their own fields.

Angelou's acknowledgment that she has imposter syndrome helps us understand how it affects people in areas other than job success. Bullying causes psychological damage to individuals, irrespective of their achievements or social status.

Case Study 6: Michelle Obama

If we take a look over Michelle Obama's journey, we discover a lot of things. She went from being a private person to being the First Lady of the United States, even though she had some doubts. In her book "Becoming," she talked about how scared she was at first when she became famous. She got tense when she thought about being watched all the time and being asked to do a lot of things.

She was honest about her worries and fears about having such a big and public part in interviews and in her own words. She was scared of the big duties that came with being First Lady and wasn't sure if she was ready for everyone to notice her.

But Michelle Obama handled the problems with class and determination, even though she had some doubts at first. Many people looked up to her and were inspired to face their fears and go after their goals by seeing how she changed over time. At first, she didn't need to feel more secure. Instead, she had to learn how to play her part and use her fame to fight for causes she cared about.

Her story is very strong because it helps people understand themselves. It shows that even the First Lady, who was very successful and cool, had doubts and checks on herself. People look up to Michelle Obama because she is honest about her path. Fears are normal, but people shouldn't let them stop them from going forward.

There's more to "Becoming" than just her life. It's also about development, bravery, and how important it is to be honest about yourself. People like Howard Schultz, Sheryl Sandberg, Indra Nooyi, Elon Musk, and Michelle Obama have told their stories, and they can teach us a lot about how to get over imposter syndrome. What they taught us that was the most important thing. The first step is to acknowledge our self-doubt. You need to understand that mistakes are normal and that failing is a chance to learn and get better. Having a desire to grow and getting help from teachers are both great ways to shift our attention from trying to be flawless to enjoying our progress.

Strategies To Combat Imposter Syndrome

Using real-world strategies is a big part of gaining control over imposter syndrome. When we think about ourselves, we may figure out the factors that make us doubt ourselves. This lets us face our bad thoughts and change them. We can feel better about ourselves when we succeed in small ways by dividing our objectives down into steps we can actually follow. We believe in ourselves more when we learn new things. Be kind to yourself when things go wrong, and accept that failure is a part of the process. This will help you feel strong and good about yourself.

Making these ideas and habits a part of our daily lives gives us the tools we need to deal with imposter syndrome. It's about using your doubt to help you grow in your personal and professional life while managing your flaws.

References

"Maya Angelou: And Still I Rise." Directed by Bob Hercules and Rita Coburn Whack, 2016.

Angelou, M. (2009). "Letter to My Daughter." Random House.

Angelou, M. (2013). "Mom & Me & Mom." Random House.

Interviews and speeches delivered by Michelle Obama, including those conducted during her time as First Lady and in subsequent public appearances. These discussions often touch upon her initial reservations and eventual growth into her role, inspiring others to face their insecurities.

Interviews with Maya Angelou, including those conducted by Oprah Winfrey and other media outlets, where she openly discussed her personal experiences and feelings of imposter syndrome.

Musk, E. (Interviews, speeches, and articles). Various media outlets, including TED Talks, CNBC, and interviews in publications like Wired and Forbes.

Nooyi, I. (Interviews, speeches, and articles). Various media outlets, including Forbes, Fortune, and Harvard Business Review.

Obama, M. (2018). "Becoming." Crown Publishing Group. Her memoir "Becoming" delves into her personal journey, including her initial apprehensions about entering the public sphere and how she navigated and embraced her role as First Lady.

Sandberg, S. (2013). "Lean In: Women, Work, and the Will

to Lead." Knopf.

Schultz, H., & Yang, D. (1999). "Pour Your Heart Into It: How Starbucks Built a Company One Cup at a Time." Hachette Books.

Chapter 10
Strategies, Recommendations, and Conclusion

Impostor syndrome goes beyond a mere feeling—it embodies the persistent belief that one must adopt a persona different from their authentic self to earn respect and assert authority. It manifests as a tendency to emulate others in leadership roles, seeking external validation and adhering to perceived norms, rather than embracing one's true, authentic self.

This phenomenon captures the internal struggle of individuals who harbor a deep-seated fear of being unmasked as inadequate or undeserving of their positions. The impostor syndrome narrative often compels individuals to perform a role dictated by external expectations rather than expressing their genuine capabilities and unique leadership style.

Rather than leading authentically, those experiencing impostor syndrome may find themselves constantly looking to others for guidance on how to be a leader, inadvertently sacrificing one's authenticity in the process. The fear of being perceived as a fraud or falling short of expectations can create a perpetual cycle of self-doubt, hindering one's ability to lead with confidence and originality.

At its core, impostor syndrome is a complex interplay of self-perception, societal expectations, and the internalized pressure to conform. It underscores the importance of recognizing and embracing one's true self, allowing for genuine leadership that stems from authenticity, confidence, and a deep understanding of one's capabilities.

To overcome impostor syndrome is to liberate oneself from the shackles of external expectations, fostering an environment where leaders can lead with authenticity and inspire others to do the same. It is a journey towards self-acceptance, acknowledging that true leadership emerges when individuals are unafraid to showcase their genuine selves, vulnerabilities, and strengths alike.

In essence, impostor syndrome prompts us to question the conventional norms of leadership, encouraging a shift towards a more inclusive, diverse, and authentic approach—one that celebrates the uniqueness of each leader and values the richness that diversity brings to the collective narrative of leadership.

In the exploration of overcoming imposter syndrome, let's compile a comprehensive list of strategies and practical implications that you can derive from this guide. Each strategy is accompanied by real-life examples to elucidate its application.

1. **Develop Self-awareness:**
   - Strategy: Gain awareness of how imposter syndrome manifests in your life.
   - Practical Implication: Maintain a journal to record instances of self-doubt and identify patterns. Recognize specific triggers that exacerbate imposter feelings.
   - Example: Regularly reflecting on your experiences and emotions allows you to pinpoint areas for personal development. For instance, noting moments of self-doubt during team meetings can lead to a better understanding of your insecurities.

2. **Accept Your Weaknesses:**
   - Strategy: Embrace vulnerability by acknowledging

and discussing your shortcomings.

- Practical Implication: Share your challenges openly with peers or mentors, fostering an environment of authenticity.
- Example: A leader admitting to struggling with time management during a team meeting creates an atmosphere where others feel comfortable acknowledging one's own struggles, thereby breaking down the stigma associated with imperfections.

3. **Set Realistic Expectations:**
- Strategy: Establish achievable goals and recognize the inevitability of making mistakes.
- Practical Implication: Break down large objectives into smaller, manageable tasks, allowing for incremental progress.
- Example: Instead of aiming for perfection in a project, focus on continuous improvement. Celebrate milestones and view setbacks as opportunities for learning and growth.

4. **Seek Mentorship and Support:**
- Strategy: Leverage guidance from mentors and build a strong support network.
- Practical Implication: Actively seek advice from experienced individuals who have overcome imposter syndrome.
- Example: Regularly consulting with a mentor who has navigated similar challenges provides valuable insights and encouragement, reinforcing your ability to overcome self-doubt.

5. **Develop a Growth Mentality:**
- Strategy: Embrace challenges as opportunities for

learning and personal development.

- Practical Implication: Shift from a fixed mindset to a growth-oriented perspective that values continuous improvement.
- Example: Viewing setbacks as chances to refine your skills fosters resilience and transforms imposter feelings into motivation for self-improvement.

6. **Celebrate Your Successes:**
   - Strategy: Acknowledge and appreciate your achievements, no matter how small.
   - Practical Implication: Maintain a success journal to document accomplishments and boost self-esteem.
   - Example: Recognizing and celebrating small victories, such as successfully leading a team meeting or completing a challenging task, reinforces a positive self-image and counters imposters' thoughts.

7. **Help Create a Friendly Environment:**
   - Strategy: Foster a workplace culture that encourages open communication, empathy, and mutual support.
   - Practical Implication: Actively engage in team-building activities and promote a sense of camaraderie.
   - Example: Initiating informal discussions within the team and providing constructive feedback creates an atmosphere where individuals feel comfortable sharing concerns, diminishing the impact of imposter syndrome.

8. **Encourage Diversity and Inclusion:**
   - Strategy: Recognize and appreciate diverse

strengths and perspectives within a team.

- Practical Implication: Actively support initiatives that promote diversity and inclusion.
- Example: Acknowledging and valuing the unique contributions of team members from different backgrounds enhances collective problem-solving and fosters a culture where everyone's skills are recognized, reducing imposter syndrome's grip on individuals.

By integrating these strategies into your life, you can cultivate a resilient mindset and create an environment that promotes personal and collective growth.

As I draw the curtains on our exploration of overcoming imposter syndrome, I aim to leave you not just informed but equipped with the tools for lasting confidence and empowerment. Throughout our journey together, I have underscored the critical importance of addressing imposter syndrome for its profound impact on personal and professional success.

Overcoming imposter syndrome is akin to unlocking a door that leads to newfound determination and purpose. This process involves a deliberate effort to recognize and dismantle patterns of self-doubt, celebrate achievements, and foster a supportive environment. By consistently implementing these actions, you not only pave the way for personal growth but also set the stage for a more fulfilling and rewarding career trajectory.

It is imperative to understand that conquering imposter syndrome is a dynamic journey, one that is entirely achievable as you navigate the intricacies of your personal experiences. The strategies outlined in this exploration provide practical and realistic ideas, inspired by real-life leaders who have grappled with similar challenges. Cultivating a growth mentality, embracing transparency about your vulnerabilities, and seeking mentorship are potent tools that can catalyze transformative change in your life.

In offering recommendations for individuals and organizations seeking assistance with imposter syndrome, I emphasize the following:

1. **Implement Training Programs**: Organizations can design and implement training programs that address imposter syndrome. These programs could include workshops, seminars, or coaching sessions to raise awareness, provide coping strategies, and foster a supportive culture.

2. **Establish Mentorship Programs**: Encourage the creation of mentorship programs within organizations, pairing experienced individuals with those who may be struggling with imposter feelings. This mentorship can provide guidance, share experiences, and offer a supportive network.

3. **Promote Open Communication**: Create an environment where open communication is not only encouraged but celebrated. This could involve regular team discussions, forums, or even anonymous platforms where individuals feel safe expressing their concerns and seeking advice.

4. **Recognize and Reward Accomplishments**: Organizations can implement recognition programs that highlight and reward individual and team accomplishments. This can help counteract imposter feelings by reinforcing the value and competence of each team member.

5. **Provide Resources for Personal Development**: Organizations can invest in resources such as training

materials, books, or counseling services to support employees in their personal development journey. This proactive approach can contribute to a healthier workplace culture.

Self-perspective checklist for readers to gauge their progress in overcoming imposter syndrome:

Self-Perspective Checklist:

1. **Self-awareness**: Am I actively identifying patterns of self-doubt and addressing them?
2. **Acceptance of Weaknesses**: Have I embraced transparency about my vulnerabilities and sought support?
3. **Realistic Expectations**: Do I set achievable goals and view mistakes as opportunities for learning?
4. **Mentorship and Support**: Have I actively sought guidance from mentors and built a strong support network?
5. **Growth Mentality**: Do I approach challenges with a mindset focused on continuous improvement?
6. **Celebration of Successes**: Do I acknowledge and celebrate my achievements, no matter how small?
7. **Contribution to a Friendly Environment**: Am I actively fostering a workplace culture that encourages open communication and support?
8. **Encouragement of Diversity and Inclusion**: Am I recognizing and appreciating diverse strengths and perspectives within my team?

Conclusion

In conclusion, I hope the insights shared in these pages serve as a roadmap for you, empowering you to confront imposter syndrome with courage and determination. Your worthiness of achievement is rooted in your capabilities. Let this understanding propel you forward on your journey, enabling you to confront self-doubt and embrace a future marked by confidence and purpose.

In our investigation of overcoming impostor syndrome, I want to have instilled in you a strong sense of confidence and empowerment. Our experience together has highlighted how important it is to address imposter syndrome for both your personal and professional success.

It's like opening a door to new determination and purpose when you recognize and overcome imposter syndrome. It entails identifying the patterns of self-doubt, acknowledging your accomplishments, and creating a welcoming and supportive atmosphere. When these actions are done consciously and regularly, they open doors to both personal development and a more rewarding career path.

It's important to keep in mind that overcoming imposter syndrome is a journey and completely achievable as you work through the complexity of your personal experiences. The tactics covered offer useful and realistic ideas and have been modeled after actual leaders who have faced similar difficulties. Develop a growth mentality, embrace honesty, and look for mentorship. These simple yet powerful strategies have the potential to change lives.

Lastly, may the knowledge and insight conveyed in these pages act as a road map for you, enabling you to face the impostor syndrome head-on with courage and determination. You are worthy of achievement because you are capable. Allow this insight to move you forward on your journey, giving you the means to face self-doubt and welcome a confident and purposeful future.

About the Author

Retired Air Force Master Sergeant | Author | CEO | Strategic Leader | Professor

Dr. Joshan A. Flowers a retired Air Force Master Sergeant, brings a wealth of experience and expertise to the table. With a distinguished military career and a passion for leadership and personal development, Dr. Flowers has become a recognized authority in the field of strategic leadership and Imposter Syndrome.

Born and raised in the vibrant city of Chicago, Dr. Flowers embarked on a journey that led to two master's degrees in public administration and management and leadership, earned from Webster University. Committed to lifelong learning and personal growth, Dr. Flowers went on to attain a Doctorate in Strategic Leadership from Liberty University, solidifying her commitment to excellence in leadership.

Having served as a Master Sergeant in the United States Air Force, Dr. Flowers culminated her service with a prestigious assignment at the Pentagon, specifically within the Joint Chiefs of Staff (J-1) division. Her experience and contributions at the highest levels of military leadership have not only honed her skills but have also granted her invaluable insights into leadership, strategy, and management.

As the Owner and CEO of Xceum Consulting and Services, Dr. Flowers leads a dynamic team of professionals who provide strategic guidance and consulting services to organizations seeking to optimize their leadership, management, and operational effectiveness. Dr. Flowers's dedication to improving organizations' performance and guiding them toward their strategic goals is at the heart of Xceum's mission.

Outside of her professional life, Dr. Flowers enjoys the enriching experiences of traveling, attending sporting events, and indulging in reading during her spare moments. The family remains a cornerstone of Dr. Flowers's life, as she is married and has two accomplished adult children.

Currently residing in Fort Washington, MD, Dr. Flowers continues to inspire and lead, shaping the path for others through her strategic leadership, consulting expertise, and commitment to personal development.

Made in the USA
Middletown, DE
15 January 2026

25065348R00068